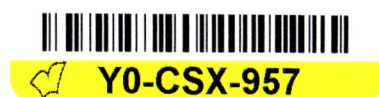

Getting Doctors to Listen

Hastings Center Studies in Ethics

A SERIES EDITED BY

Mark J. Hanson and Daniel Callahan

This series of books, published by The Hastings Center and Georgetown University Press, examines ethical issues in medicine and the life sciences. Established in 1969, The Hastings Center, located in Briarcliff Manor, New York, is an independent, nonprofit, and nonpartisan research organization. The work of the Center is mainly carried out through research projects, the publication of the *Hastings Center Report* and *IRB: A Review of Human Subjects Research*, and numerous workshops, conferences, lectures, and consultations. The **Hastings Center Studies in Ethics** series brings the ongoing research of The Hastings Center to a wider audience.

Getting Doctors to Listen
Ethics and Outcomes Data in Context

EDITED BY
Philip J. Boyle

GEORGETOWN UNIVERSITY PRESS / WASHINGTON, D.C.

Georgetown University Press, Washington, D.C. 20007
© 1998 by Georgetown University Press. All rights reserved.
Printed in the United States of America
10 9 8 7 6 5 4 3 2 1   1998
THIS VOLUME IS PRINTED ON ACID-FREE ∞ OFFSET BOOK PAPER

Library of Congress Cataloging-in-Publication Data

Getting doctors to listen : ethics and outcomes data in context /
  edited by Philip J. Boyle.
      p.   cm.—(Hastings Center studies in ethics)
    Includes bibliographical references (p.   ).
    1. Medicine—Decision making—Moral and ethical aspects.
  2. Outcome assessment (Medical care)—Moral and ethical aspects.
  3. Medical protocols—Moral and ethical aspects. 4. Physicians—
  Professional ethics.   I. Boyle, Philip.   II. Series.
  R723.5.G48   1998
  174'.2—dc21   97-9533
  ISBN 0-87840-654-9 (cloth)

Contents

Preface   vii

PART I: OVERVIEW AND CONTEXT OF
MORAL OBSTACLES   1

    PHILIP J. BOYLE AND DANIEL CALLAHAN
Physicians' Use of Outcomes Data: Moral Conflicts and
Potential Resolutions   3

    RUTH S. HANFT
Health Technology Assessment in the 1990s   21

    PAUL J. EDELSON
Clinical Practice Guidelines: A Historical Perspective on Their
Origins and Significance   31

PART II: OUTCOMES DATA   39

    JUDITH WILSON ROSS
Practice Guidelines: Texts in Search of Authority   41

    LARRY CULPEPPER AND JANE SISK
The Development of Practice Guidelines: A Case Study of
Otitis Media with Effusion   71

    GERT JAN VAN DER WILT AND PIETER F. DE VRIES ROBBÉ
The Quest for the Trial to End All Trials: The Case of
Technology Assessment and Management of Glue Ear   86

DONALD J. MURPHY
Guideline Glitches: Measurements, Money, and Malpractice   100

SUSAN E. BELL
Technology Assessment, Outcomes Data, and Social Context: The Case of Hormone Therapy   111

SUSAN E. KELLY AND BARBARA A. KOENIG
"Rescue" Technologies following High-Dose Chemotherapy for Breast Cancer: How Social Context Shapes the Assessment of Innovative, Aggressive, and Lifesaving Medical Technologies   126

DICK WILLEMS
Outcomes, Guidelines, and Implementation in France, the Netherlands, and Great Britain   153

PART III: ETHICAL CONSIDERATIONS: THE RESOLVABLE AND THE INTRACTABLE   165

FRED GIFFORD
Outcomes Research and Practice Guidelines: Upstream Issues and Epistemological Issues   167

ROBERT M. VEATCH
Technology Assessment: Inevitably a Value Judgment   180

JAMES LINDEMANN NELSON
Clinical Judgment versus Outcomes Research?   196

SANDRA J. TANENBAUM
Say the Right Thing: Communication and Physician Accountability in the Era of Medical Outcomes   204

Contributors   225

Index   227

Preface

The story told in this book emerged from Dan Callahan's hunch that a significant trend within health care—the implementation of outcomes data and practice guidelines—might simply stall from resistance to the data by its physician-users. Careful listening to physicians indicated that they provide many moral sounding reasons (e.g., "My patient understood the recommendations but wants some other intervention") for setting aside recommendations that were associated with outcomes data and practice guidelines. Dan hypothesized that this moral resistance could undercut the outcomes movement; alternatively, if the moral resistance was identified and addressed, then this could improve acceptance of outcomes data. The Agency for Health Care Policy and Research (AHCPR) of the National Institutes of Health concurred that this hypothesis needed to be explored, so it funded a two-year study at The Hastings Center. Terry Shannon of AHCPR was particularly instrumental in providing direction and support for carrying out the project.

The attempt to identify and understand the moral reasons given by physicians resistant to using outcomes data required the participation of dozens of physicians from four sites around the country. Not all of the countless individuals can be thanked here for the hours they donated by participating in focus groups and research meetings. The project members who have contributed to this volume are visible; however, other project members who nurtured these ideas require special thanks. Foremost, the advice of Sandy Tanenbaum was seminal for thinking through the ideas articulated in this book.

In addition to Dan Callahan, other colleagues at the Center provided important critique and support for teasing out the medical details and philosophical issues, including, Joe Fins, MD, Jim and Hilde Nelson, Bette Crigger and Bruce Jennings. Moreover several projects members made the focus groups possible at the sites, most especially Wilmer Rutt, MD, Jane Gerety, Susan Hill, MD, Jeff Brensilver, MD, and Douglas Owens, MD.

Other participants who contributed to the project include: Renée Anspach, Marianne Baird, Eric J. Cassell, MD, Alan R. Fleischman, MD, Cornelia Fleming, Thomas Glenn, MD, Sidney Goldstein, MD, Hank Greely, Ichiro Kawachi, MD, Elizabeth Lane, MD, Nathan Levin, MD, Michael Massanari,

MD, Bruce McCarthy, MD, David Miller, MD, Elizabeth Mort, MD, Kathryn Moseley, MD, George Nolan, MD, Emanual Rivers, MD, Jeffrey Stier, MD, Frank Stockdale, MD., John D. Tracy, MD, Richard Ward, MD, and Alan J. Weisbard.

Last, but by no means least, Janet Bower, Jennifer Stuber, and Marna Howarth of the Center provided the hidden but essential support to get this book out. To all these colleagues I am forever grateful.

Getting Doctors to Listen

PART I: Overview and Context of Moral Obstacles

Philip J. Boyle and Daniel Callahan
Physicians' Use of Outcomes Data: Moral Conflicts and Potential Resolutions

Ruth S. Hanft
Health Technology Assessment in the 1990s

Paul J. Edelson
Clinical Practice Guidelines: A Historical Perspective on Their Origins and Significance

Philip J. Boyle and Daniel Callahan

Physicians' Use of Outcomes Data: Moral Conflicts and Potential Resolutions

Background

Is clinical medicine best thought of as a science or an art?[1] The question is an old one, now given a fresh life by the powerful movement to develop outcomes data and practice guidelines. The assumption behind the movement is that a combination of good data and well-crafted guidelines will save money and more effectively serve patient care. It is an assumption that is heavily biased toward construing medicine more as science than as art.

Such a bias does not always sit well with practicing physicians. Sinclair Lewis caught the flavor of physicians' unease in a conversation between two doctors in his now classic novel *Arrowsmith,* written in 1924:

> Doctor, do you find you can do much with asthma? Well now, Doctor, just in confidence, I'm going to tell you something that may strike you as funny, but I believe foxes' lungs are just fine for asthma, and T.B. too. I told that to a Sioux City pulmonary specialist one time and he laughed at me—said it wasn't scientific . . . I said "But I get results, and that's what I'm looking for." . . . I swear I believe most of these damn' alleged scientists could learn a whale of a lot from the plain country practitioners, let me tell you!

In a recent study carried out by The Hastings Center, we sought to study this time-worn issue in the context of the renewed effort to influence physicians' behavior by providing them with better science and helpful guidelines for their clinical practice. What is new, perhaps unique, about the issue and found in the outcomes enterprise is a shift from physician reliance on traditional biomedical reasoning to a reliance on probabilistic statistical reasoning.[2] We had noted that, for all of the technical skills being deployed to develop good data, something seemed missing. While some research has examined changing physician behavior with a mix of techniques,[3] there has been practically no effort to explore the way physicians respond to data and guidelines that present a moral challenge or threat to practitioners' values and clinical experience. There is surely some evidence that in many cases data and guidelines improve the process of care,[4] but also evidence that in other cases—advanced cardiac life support[5] and the management of chest pain, for instance[6]—guidelines are often resisted or ignored.[7] If the entire outcomes enterprise is to be successful, it will be necessary to understand better the way in which the intended users of its products will respond to, and use or not use, what is pressed upon them.[8]

Our study tried to begin that effort by unearthing the objections, hesitations, and uncertainties physicians are likely to feel—but not always to openly express—in the face of data and guidelines challenging their own practice. We were in particular stimulated by the fact that, in our initial exchanges, many physicians expressed their concerns in the language of morality or something close to it: "The data is tainted"; or "I agree with the data, but I owe it to my patients to follow their wishes"; or "I would violate my clinical integrity if I followed the guidelines"; or "It is just too uncomfortable to talk with patients about these matters, and besides, I just don't have time."

While by no means are all objections and hesitations moral in character, as we will develop, moral concerns seem at the heart of much resistance and thus became the focus of our study. By a "moral" problem we mean an objection or hesitation based on a physician's feeling or belief that to act on some new data or to change his or her behavior in response to the guidelines would threaten his or her professional integrity—his or her medical ethic—and thus pose dangers to, or inflict direct harm upon, their patients. This kind of concern often overlapped worries about legal liability, financial incentives, and the scientific validity of the data. They were no less part of a common physician concern to find the best way of balancing outcomes data, clinical experience, and patient requests or demands.

The aim of our study was to identify the moral and related problems of physicians when confronted with outcomes data and practice guidelines, to assess the merits of their concerns, and to propose some ways of responding to them. If the objections, worries, and hesitations can be better understood, it might be possible to design more effective guidelines, to develop more useful data, and to advance the cause of good outcomes assessment. This position assumes—for the purposes of exposition—that the implementation of outcomes data and practice guidelines will on balance produce more good practice than bad.

Before proceeding directly to the results of our study, however, it may be helpful to say a brief word about the generation of outcomes data and the development of practice guidelines. A fair degree of confusion and skepticism seems common among practicing physicians, based, at least in part, on the complexity and variety of the ways in which outcomes data are generated. Outcomes data are produced by several means[9]—clinical trials, insurance claims databases, and meta-analysis, for example—and they are provided to clinicians in ways ranging from presentations of the raw data alone to their incorporation in practice guidelines. This variety in the means of presentation seems itself a source of physicians' uncertainty. That uncertainty can become all the more pronounced when a technology or therapy is assessed by a number of different means, often over an extended period of time with divergent, sometimes contradictory, results. That some data are presented in an ostensibly value-free way but in fact seem to carry with them a tacit recommendation, can create suspicion. When data that are themselves debated and debatable are used to undergird practice guidelines, then the suspicion is likely to be heightened. It is not our task here to assess the value and validity of outcomes studies or practice guidelines. We only want to note that physician concern or skepticism about these can stimulate or reinforce clinicians' moral anxieties—many of which might exist even in the absence of hesitations about the value and validity of the data or the guidelines given them.

Yet there is also no doubt that greater efforts to improve the quality of the data, to find consistent ways of presenting it, to reveal openly all sources of financial support for the studies, and to make use of would be clinician users in the design of outcomes studies and the clinical guidelines would help to minimize many such problems. No less helpful would be a lively awareness on the part of those interested in adoption of outcomes data that physician response is likely to be a complex mixture of many factors. It will include an assessment of the data, the authority on which the data or guidelines are presented, the subspecialty of the user, the nature of the disease to be treated, the kind of intervention recommended, and the affected patient population. At all times it is necessary to keep in mind that there has never been a satisfactory resolution, accepted by all, of the long-standing debate on the proper balance between the science and the art of medicine. If contemporary doctors do not talk exactly like those in *Arrowsmith,* many will nonetheless feel quite at home with the sentiments expressed in the dialogue we quoted in our opening paragraph.

Method

To get a better understanding of the range of hesitations that clinicians seem to have about outcomes data and practice guidelines, our interdisciplinary research group conducted interviews with individual physicians and organized a series of structured discussions with groups of physicians from a variety of different institutions. Our aim was simply to identify the kinds of conflicts, moral as well as related clinical, that physicians feel. For our purposes, it was not necessary to break down or classify the types of expressed conflicts by type of institution, or subspecialty, or age, or other sociological characteristics. We sought only to identify the kinds of felt problems, concluding our survey when it became clear that we had reached the point of repetitive and familiar responses. Out of this process, which elicited a heterogeneous response, we then classified the moral problems into the most common categories.

The clinical-staff discussions were held at four diverse medical centers: a midwestern inner-city HMO, a West Coast teaching and research hospital, a southern tertiary care institution, and a northeastern community hospital. We sought to raise the relevant issues in the context of a range of technologies and therapies to encompass a variety of available outcomes data and practice guidelines, a range of subspecialties, a variety of interventions (e.g., drugs, preventive strategies, surgery), a range of settings in which the technologies or therapies are used (e.g., acute care and clinics), and a breadth of patients served (e.g., young and old, male and female). Ten technologies were chosen for examination: thrombolytic therapies (streptokinase vs. tissue plasminogen activator [t-Pa]), hormone replacement therapy (HRT), prostate-specific antigen (PSA), ear tubes for otitis media, smoking-cessation therapies, cholesterol screening, treatment of low-birthweight babies, and autologous bone marrow transplantation for advanced breast cancer (ABMT).

Concerning the specific technologies, we wanted to know: (1) Were the clinicians aware of the available outcomes data and/or practice guidelines? (2) Did their institutions have an official policy on the use of the technologies? (3) Did the physicians take seriously (e.g., consider and adopt) the data and/or guidelines, and if their institution had a specific policy, did physicians take that seriously? (4) Did the physicians pattern their own behavior on the outcomes data and/or guidelines or on their institutional policies? (5) What kinds of difficulties, hesitations, and problems did the physicians have with the outcomes data and the available practice guidelines. We report here primarily on question 5.

Results

The moral and quasi-moral physician objections, worries, and hesitations that we discovered broke down into three broad categories: (1) skepticism about the source, reliability, and objectivity of outcomes data, including the validity of inferences drawn from the data to construct practice guidelines; (2) objections or hesitations based not on the reliability of the data or guideline recommendations but on contrary patient preferences, clinical experience, and legal worries; and (3) tacit motivation, rarely stated but apparent in the sociological literature and/or admitted hesitatingly by physicians. Within these three broad categories, we focused specifically on seven particular worries: biased and defective methodology, unwarranted inferences drawn from the data, patient preferences, clinical experience, unobservable benefits and harms, legal liability, and additional tacit motivations.

We will now summarize the objections and worries we heard and then offer some comments on their validity and the ways in which many of the objections might be minimized, even if not entirely eliminated, in the future.

Biased and Defective Methodology

While by no means universal, we found considerable skepticism about outcomes studies, based on a perceived or assumed bias on the part of those who carried out the studies or based on criticism of the methodology used. We did not ourselves attempt to determine the validity of this skepticism; we only report its existence. We found, for instance, considerable doubt about the reliability of the GUSTO II megatrial,[10] with its impressive trial population of 40,000 but financed by a biotechnology company with a vested interest in the outcomes. This doubt existed despite the fact that there were no serious methodological criticisms of the study by research experts; it seemed, instead, to be based on an assumption that, inevitably, financial interests must have had a serious influence on the study. More generally, there seems to be a widespread skepticism, or something close to it, about outcomes studies, as if—whatever the specific evidence to back up such judgments—they must be permeated with bias. It would, therefore, be irresponsible to change clinical practice based on data of that kind.

Yet given the evidence that physicians do sometimes change their behavior on the basis of outcomes data and practice guidelines, it is evident that not all physicians are cynical or skeptical about methodological bias or that they change their behavior anyway. But it was a common enough objection to make clear that as much care as possible must be taken to avoid both the reality and the appearance of bias or conflict of interest. The authority behind the outcomes data or practice guidelines is no less important an issue. That some outcomes analyses are based on one kind of data (e.g., megatrials), while other data come from administrative databases, creates doubt about the comparative reliability and authority of the data. When experts themselves argue about the comparative validity of different kinds of data, it is hardly surprising that many physicians become skeptical of the entire enterprise: their own experience, or that of their local colleagues, can seem much more compelling. Given the fact that most physicians will not have the specialized training, much less the time, needed to evaluate outcomes studies, the way in which such studies are presented will make a considerable difference in their acceptance. They must not only be authoritative and unbiased; they must *appear* that way.

The methodological objections often focused on the reliability of the sample used, carelessly organized randomized clinical trials, and mistakenly drawn conclusions from the research data. As with the charge of bias, it frequently appeared that there was little basis for the skepticism—it represented a kind of emotional reaction. But in other cases—as with some practice guidelines for the treatment of middle-ear infections in children[11]—there appeared to be a stronger justification for the skepticism. In the latter case, moreover, the perceived problems with the data quickly generated a more wholesale set of suspicions about the development of otitis media guidelines: that one group of subspecialists had dominated the guidelines committee, that it used faulty reasoning in arriving at its conclusions, and that it biased and colored the way it presented its own findings and recommendations.[12] Suspicion, it seems, can be like a spreading ink blot, needing little to give it rapid momentum.

For the most part, problems of this kind seem correctable, particularly by strong efforts to ensure the consistency and integrity of the guideline development process. Standardization of that process—pressed by the Agency for Health Care Research and Policy, many professional organizations, and the AMA—could help considerably here.[13] Nonetheless, it appeared to us that many physicians, challenged by new data and guidelines, will continue to be skeptical, with or without adequate justification; and since they will rarely be in a position to mount their own studies, they are likely to pay more attention to their suspicions than to the evidence. Of course, that will be particularly true when the data or guidelines threaten their own beliefs and experience. Once again, we are brought back to the tension between the science and the art of medicine. Many physicians will continue to feel that, when faced with a conflict of this kind, they owe it to their professional integrity and their patients to trust their clinical experience rather than outcomes data or guidelines.

Hidden Values

A problem similar to, but not quite the same as, allegations of biased research is the charge that outcomes data and guidelines reflect hidden, unacknowledged values. This appears most apparent (rightly or wrongly) to physicians who feel that these unacknowledged values go counter to their own. In the case of very low birthweight babies, for example, different studies have interpreted the same facts differently and implicitly recommended a variety of courses of action. One study, for instance, assessed survivability as a good outcome,[14] while other studies considered only survival without devastating neurological deficits to be a good result.[15] Such differences evidently reflect the different values of the researchers and/or those who make use of the available outcomes data. The physicians themselves, moreover, bring their own values to their reading of the data. Some physicians we interviewed claimed that even a 1 percent chance of survival, whatever the neurological devastation, was a good outcome. Many nurses, by contrast, felt that the pursuit of survival at all costs is unacceptable.

The problem of hidden or implicit values is not all that easy to respond to. In the nature of the case, practice guidelines based on some particular data set (or combination of sets) will be based on some values or other; they cannot, by definition, be value-free.[16] Moreover, it is often the case that even when specific practice recommendations are not attached to outcomes data, they may seem implicit in the data or the way the data are presented. Only data that are presented as outcomes probabilities only, with no hint of a value stance toward the data, are likely to qualify as value-free. Hence, one strategy to deal with the allegation of a value bias, or suspicion that it is tacitly present, would be a scrupulous effort to remove any hint of value predilections and to present the data in a way that left it entirely up to the users to apply their own values. This option might relieve the suspicions of many physicians, but it would leave the outcomes movement falling well short of the expectation that it will change physician behavior when that seems necessary. If physicians are not nudged by the data together with some different values, there is no reason to believe they will give up their own long-held values; they will simply interpret the new data in light of their own values.

Another option is self-evident. If guideline recommendations are to be made, why not simply admit, explicate, and justify the values inherent in the guidelines? This seems to us a perfectly reasonable, even preferable, option. Those presenting the guidelines would then be free to attempt by rational persuasion to make their own values seem compelling and to show that they are the most rational values in light of the available outcomes data. It will then be understood that the physicians for whom the guidelines are intended may well have different values and that the purpose of the guidelines is to directly challenge them. As long as guidelines are understood to be recommendations only, not inflexible demands, this should be an acceptable procedure, trying in effect to open a dialogue between the values of those who produced the guidelines and those who will use them. It seems also important to note here that if the guidelines have been well developed, their organizers will have done their homework—understanding, even as they develop their guidelines, what the likely value objections will be. They should, that is, know the values of their intended audience and then devise ways of presenting their data and recommendations that grapple directly with those values.

Patient Preferences

A significant proportion of the physicians we interviewed cited patient preferences as a determinative reason not to abide by the recommendations for action associated with outcomes data. The tension was most evident in cases where outcomes data predict that an intervention will be no more effective than doing nothing, but physicians believe patient preferences for an action provide an overriding justification for intervening anyway. Some parents of children with otitis media demanded ear tubes as opposed to watchful waiting, for example, even though the data clearly showed there is overall no difference in outcomes—their children fit exactly into the population for whom watchful waiting would have been as effective as inserting ear tubes. In other cases, by contrast, some physicians who believed findings that an intervention would have an effect and agreed with the findings' recommendations for action nonetheless did not proceed when faced with patient resistance, such as smoking cessation and hormone replacement therapy (HRT).

In the face of some uncertainty about the long- and short-term effects of certain kinds of hormone replacement therapy,[17] for example, physicians would defer to women who wanted to avoid what patients considered harmful effects, such as bleeding and weight gain. Of course, the willingness of a physician to grant patients' desires was complicated by the physician's own professional interpretation of data and assessment of risk.[18] Unlike some bone marrow transplant specialists who, in the face of little evidence of what the effect on advanced breast cancer will be, were willing to follow women's wishes,[19] some oncologists, believing they knew what the effects would be and how to value those effects, viewed the risks of bone marrow therapy as so greatly exceeding the benefits for women that they refused to provide it.[20] The complexity of physicians' reasons for following or resisting outcomes data does not, however, undermine the fact that patient preferences are a potent ingredient for physician moral resistance to outcomes data.

Physician deference to patient preferences might practically, if not morally, be responded to by institutional constraints on the physician, such as financial incentives for compliance by decreasing reimbursement in the face of failure to comply. The moral problem would not be so easily skirted, however, in situations that permit the intervention when private financing is available. If institutional policies permit and the patient can pay for it, however, the course of least physician resistance is deferring to patient requests. This course of action suggests that recommendations that follow from outcomes data are just that, recommendations and not mandates. But a moral tension is created: patients are left as the final arbiters about any treatment to select (even those with little or no effect), but those who produce outcomes data have expectations that physicians (and patients) will implement recommendations based on those data. Officially deferring to patient wishes might eliminate physician resistance but simultaneously move the debate to a broader social question about whether and how to effect implementation of outcomes data recommendations.

Another course of action would be to remove the choice from physicians entirely. If the outcomes data clearly supported a specific course of action, but one that physicians were uncomfortable implementing, the moral problem could be shifted to one of social enforcement. Smoking cessation offers the clearest example. Many physicians show reluctance to press for smoking cessation in any vigorous way, for moral or practical reasons. Strategies for implementing smoking cessation have not been left to physicians alone, however. A host of other effective social measures (e.g., social pressure, antismoking laws) have been adopted.[21] Where physicians' actions play a significant and direct role in implementing recommendations that follow from outcomes data, studies have been conducted to identify social features that disrupt implementation of recommendations.[22] While these studies may help to stimulate higher rates of use of the valued interventions on the part of physicians, they leave untouched the question of whether society should be promoting some outcomes over patients' preferences. Also untouched is the moral issue of how far the physician should go in persuading or inducing patients to comply with recommendations that follow from outcomes data. If they are supported, say, by HMO policy, this may be easy to do in cases where patient desires will not merit coverage for the patient. It will be harder when the patient is willing to pay out of pocket.

Clinical Experience

Some physicians—especially those who had years of clinical experience or specialty training concerning the technology currently studied—frequently did not directly dispute the reliability and validity of the outcomes data but resisted the associated recommendations. They cited instead the superiority of their own clinical experience and knowledge. The clearest example was in the case of endarterectomies in this study's preliminary research. Vascular surgeons and neurologists agreed with recommendations based on outcomes data that only a level of 70 percent or greater of arterial stenosis warranted an endarterectomy.[23] An interviewed vascular surgeon, who had performed thousands of endarterectomies, commonly performed the surgery on patients well below the stenosis level. She cited her professional clinical judgment to justify that practice.

Her response was not atypical and was encountered with many other technologies as well. It was, once again, a reflection of the claim of medicine as an art over medicine as a science. The reasoning of the physicians played upon two issues. One of them is that there is a difference between statistical outcomes in general for a class of patients and what might be effective with a particular patient. Outcomes assessments are probabilistic; they do not guarantee what might be efficacious in individual cases. A second issue turned on the belief that clinical experience can discern and take account of more evidence than encompassed within the scope of outcomes research. At the heart of the complaint against "cookbook medicine" is the belief that it runs roughshod over clinical experience and the uniqueness of individual cases.

These objections are not easily pushed aside. They directly express a long and deep tradition in medicine, and they play as well upon the gap between statistical patient populations and specific patients. One way of ameliorating the struggle here would be to think of practice guidelines working along a continuum in the promotion of compliance. At one end, outcomes research could be developed to persuade physicians rationally to prefer its judgments over clinical knowledge. Practice guidelines, for example, could include explicit reasons why their normative requirements do not allow for resistance (e.g., it is too inefficient for the system, or when resource are scarce, it is less permissible). Strong disincentives could be created to enforce the guidelines (e.g., by penalizing salary for practicing outside a reasonable range). These pragmatic solutions miss, however, the troubling moral problem that claims of clinical experience raise—the need of physicians to act in a way that manifests their medical integrity, which has historically also included a conscientious reliance on their clinical experience.

At the other end of the spectrum, far removed from direct coercion of physicians to follow guidelines, would be a twofold effort: to work more closely with clinicians in devising the guidelines in the first place, taking account of their experience; and to allow physicians, on a principled basis, to deviate from the recommendations for action in the practice guidelines. This approach would accept the legitimacy of individualized physician judgments with particular patients. Some clinical choices might be ruled out altogether, but beyond that there would be room for discretion. At some point, however, if the findings of the outcomes data are strong and compelling, there may be no reasonable course other than to restrict choice and override the claims of experience or patient uniqueness. At some point, science will have to push aside art, however unpleasant this may be.

Unobservable Benefits and Harms

A few physicians resisted the outcomes data because they understood the data answered some questions, but not *their* question; consequently, the data were less significant to their practice. With technologies where physicians can not directly observe the harm of not intervening, or the benefits of intervention (where there is a time gap between the intervention and observable effects), or physicians do not sense an immediate great risk to the patient, physicians' responses suggested that outcomes data were less important. In the case of cholesterol screening to identify patients at higher risk of cardiac illness, physicians who followed the recommendations derived from outcomes data for screening and necessary treatment would never be certain of their successes, only their failures of not intervening early enough.[24] Likewise for smoking cessation counseling, physicians knew only in epidemiological terms, and not in tangible terms, whether their intervention was successful. In the case of autologous bone marrow transplant, the professional training of the oncologist and transplant surgeons provided opposite views of risk, the former unwilling to risk that a patient might die from the therapy, and the latter unwilling to risk the death of the patient from lack of therapy, even in the absence of good data about its effectiveness.

The case of t-Pa and streptokinase adds an odd twist to the probability that physicians will see the results from acting on outcomes data. At one site, physicians claimed there was not enough statistical difference in the outcomes data for them to follow the implicit recommendations—and growing standard of practice—to prefer t-Pa. The tie-breaking value for these physicians was that using the less expensive streptokinase was of financial benefit for their institution. Physicians commented that when they use less expensive therapies they were aware that additional services would be made available and this perception of less cost and more service was a motivating factor. At another site, however, where fee-for-service medicine was practiced, a physician noted that even if cost had been a relevant part of the outcomes assessment (and it was not), it would have had little bearing on practice at that institution; its physicians, it was claimed, do not take account of cost. They almost exclusively used t-PA because of its perceived marginal benefit (based on the GUSTO II trial) of reducing mortality risk.

Some steps could be taken to respond to physician hesitation here. Those who develop and disseminate the data might publish the results with cues designed to assist physicians to imagine the risks for the patient of not taking seriously the data or might find ways to highlight the relationship between statistics about outcomes and outcomes for particular, identifiable patients. Alternatively, those who develop and disseminate outcomes data might resign themselves to the fact that physicians will more likely set aside data when the effects of following the data are unobservable to the physician. Physicians are more likely to refrain from the recommended action if they do not see a connection between an intervention and an outcome. This alternative accentuates the need for observable impact, which is not necessarily provided by outcomes data. Outcomes data provide a population perspective, often difficult for physicians to observe. Physicians are faced with a dilemma to either prefer the outcomes data in almost blind obedience based on the authority of the producers or to resist them, and both options are cause for moral concern.

Fear of Liability

Physicians commonly perceived threats of legal liability for either following or not following guideline recommendations.[25] In some cases where physicians agreed with and felt compelled to follow the normative conclusions of the outcomes research, they also believed they could be sued for following too rigidly the outcomes research recommendations. Without specific evidence they thought recent court cases, especially associated with managed care mandating that a physician follow outcomes research recommendations, would lead to the physician being successfully sued. In an odd twist at the HMO site, physicians expressed comfort in not providing t-Pa even though the regional practice was to prefer t-Pa over streptokinase. Physicians felt protected in preferring streptokinase over t-Pa because it was the standard of care within the HMO.

The pervasive physician fear of legal liability is a substantial obstacle to the use of outcomes data, but it is not based on any solid evidence of actual legal risk. At present, it is unclear whether, and to what extant, physicians will be held liable for following or not following outcomes data and associated practice guidelines.[26] In the era of managed care it is likely that only several years from today will it be clearer whether, and under what circumstances, physicians should be concerned about legal liability. It would be cavalier to dismiss physician worries about liability, but dangerous to allow fear of liability to paralyze the outcomes movement, especially when we know that some outcomes data demonstrate that some medical practice is harmful to patients.

One step to overcome this obstacle is for outcomes data to include explicitly, as part of subsequent recommendation, a description of what legal harms are likely to be incurred by following or not following the data.

Tacit Motivation and Unarticulated Resistance

Our study had to cope with three pervasive phenomena, none of them easy to pin down or to verify. One of them stemmed from the common charges that some physicians leveled against others: that their colleagues' stated reasons for resisting outcomes data and guidelines should not be believed, that their real motives were profit, ego, ignorance, or whatever. Another phenomenon was a difficulty in taking seriously some of the objections offered: they seemed to be mere rationalizations. Still another phenomenon, the most elusive, was that of local pressures, mores, and social dynamics. In the structured interviews, some physicians forthrightly admitted that in some cases resistance to outcomes data was subterfuge or semiconscious rationalization. A few physicians reported that outcomes data were resisted and an alternative course of action chosen for reasons of ego—to look smart in front of colleagues or patients. Not much can probably be done about that kind of thing.

But the outcomes movement needs to pay careful attention to tacit social forces that correlate well with the levels and kinds of professional training. Older specialists, citing clinical expertise, more frequently ignored the recommendations (e.g., endarterectomies) than did newly trained physicians. The latter were more likely to defer to authority, to take the outcomes data seriously, and to adopt guideline recommendations. In the case of ABMT, some oncologists who specialized in bone marrow transplant were willing to put patients at high risk, in part motivated by their professional training, whereas oncologists who had not specialized in bone marrow transplants were resistant. Some psychiatrists mentioned that a principle to "learn one drug and use it well" was the motivation for psychiatrists trained in an earlier era to resist outcomes data and to continue prescribing drugs recommended at the time of their training.

Economic motivation was at times explicitly or implicitly a source of resistance. Some physicians claimed that the outcomes data carry normative conclusions that prefer cost-cutting to quality of care. In several cases, including low-birthweight babies, ABMT, and ear tubes, this was a salient stated cause for physician resistance. More commonly reported, at the opposite end of the spectrum, was motivation based on economic gain as a formidable source of resistance to implementing outcomes data. In several cases, most notably those that required extensive physician-patient interaction, such as smoking cessation counseling, physicians were more likely not to adhere to the recommendations because it was not in their financial interests to provide lengthy, costly, time-consuming counseling. In other cases, such as the placement of ear tubes for otitis media, it was in the financial interests of the ENT we interviewed to provide more costly procedures and to avoid recommendations about watchful waiting. Even though for some general practitioners there was no direct financial compensation for not following the recommendations, they received indirect benefit through referrals and professional reciprocity.

Convenience, although rarely explicit, was described by some interviewed as motivation to resist outcomes data recommendations for action. In the case of thrombolytics, in an institution that had clear institutional recommendations for streptokinase, emergency room physicians used neither streptokinase nor t-Pa but instead used aminase because it was believed to be more convenient and efficacious during transport to another hospital. Physicians also did not want to be bothered to carry out the recommendation of the outcomes researchers if doing so required too much uncompensated care, the patient would predictably not be compliant, or the recommended intervention was distasteful. In the case of smoking cessation therapy, some younger physicians claimed, as a basis of not following institutional guidelines based on outcomes data, that it was someone else's responsibility. Further exploration revealed that the resistance was in part a function of the fact that time did not permit extensive counseling for less urgent items. In the case of HRT, some male primary care physicians said that the entire intervention was inconvenient.

In the estimation of our research group, the tacit motivations for resistance (e.g., conflicts of interest, convenience, discomfort) are moral flaws endemic to any profession and difficult to respond to. Some of them have been addressed in the business ethics literature; for example, keeping incentives at arm's length from the practitioner or promoting institutional excellence that does not substitute convenience for patients' real needs. Resistance arising from these kinds of motivation should be noted, but it is unlikely that a system responsible for the dissemination and implementation of outcomes data can respond in any useful way.

Conclusions and Reflections

The causes of moral resistance to outcomes data and practice guidelines can be responded to by considering the claims individually and by devising overall strategies to improve implementation. First and foremost, the need for physicians to act with a medical ethic of integrity must not be underestimated, especially by those interested in the dissemination and adoption of outcomes data. It is important that physicians believe they are acting in a morally justifiable way, consistent with the traditions of good clinical medicine and medical ethics. At a minimum, this means avoiding a cookbook medicine, on the one hand, and unscientific clinical judgment, on the other.

Second, it must be kept in mind that the project's interviews and interdisciplinary discussion point to a great heterogeneity in the kinds of moral resistance of physicians to outcomes data and practice guidelines. Some physicians are readily compliant, others resist at first and then accede, and still others totally set aside recommended actions. Initially our project focused only on physicians' resistance; but both physicians' resistance to and their acceptance of outcomes data should create moral concern. For physicians who are by and large compliant and increasingly pressed by managed care organizations to adopt the recommendations associated with managed care, those interested in outcomes data adoption need to give some thought to aspects of clinical experience that might be unfortunately abandoned in the push for implementing outcomes data. For physicians who are resistant to implementing outcomes data, in part out of a concern to avoid a cookbook kind of medicine, there is the possibility that physician discretion will reign untrammeled and any benefits to be produced by the outcomes movement will be lost.

In the case of physicians who either too readily adopt, too readily resist, or resist guideline recommendations for action, it is reasonable to wonder whether there are some general procedural considerations for all parties in the process. For the developers of outcomes data, it is imperative to include practicing clinician participation in all aspects of the outcomes data research, for example, to ensure that physicians' sensitivities and concerns are addressed as much as is feasible. It is no less important that they have a hand in fashioning practice guidelines. For physicians, it is reasonable to expect them to seriously read outcomes literature, either to avoid rejecting out of hand all outcomes data or to avoid being so compliant as to blindly follow the recommendations of others. If, after seriously considering the outcomes data, they find significant discrepancy between the recommendations associated with outcomes data and their own desires, then conscientious physicians would need to explore further the reasons for their resistance, some of which might be defensible and others not. Self-examination might make physicians aware that some reasoning is indefensible, but no amount of self-examination will help physicians through some old moral questions, such as whether, when all previous examination of motivation has been exhausted, physicians should prefer their own clinical experience to the recommendations associated with outcomes data. Those who produce outcomes data, and those who want to promote use of such data, must give serious attention to how physicians should decide in these cases, and make explicit one way or the other which course of action clinicians should pursue. A first, and difficult, step toward this goal will be standardization and professional agreement on the moral and scientific force that outcomes data should have. Given the unresolved conflict over the importance of physician discretion, it seems premature on the part of those who manage outcomes data (e.g., managed care organizations) to require full and unquestioned compliance with recommendations.

We are brought back to our starting point. Is medicine science or art? The obvious answer is that it is both, as it has always been—and that the real question is how to find the right balance between them. The outcomes assessment and practice guidelines movement has the same problem, though with a clear bias in favor of the scientific resolution of clinical dilemmas where that is possible. But great care is needed here. The moral objections some physicians voice suggest, upon further analysis, that the present science of medicine needs to be augmented with other kinds of considerations, that, for example, information a skilled physician can observe in a moment of clinical judgment needs to be added to some scientific data. This does not unequivocally prove that medicine is an art, but it certainly calls for a humility about the state of our present science.

NOTES

1. This article was prepared for The Hastings Center Project "Technology Assessment: Uses, Context, and Interpretation," funded by the Agency for Health Care Policy and Research (AHCPR) grant 5 RO1 HS06688-02.

2. S. J. Tanenbaum, "Knowing and Acting in Medical Practice: The Epistemological Politics of Outcomes Research," *Journal of Health Politics, Policy, and Law* 19, no. 1 (Spring 1994): 27–44.

3. B. S. Mittman, X. Tonesk, P. D. Jacobson, "Implementing Clinical Practice Guidelines: Social Influence Strategies and Practitioner Behavior Change," *Quality Review Bulletin* 18 no. 12 (1992): 413–22; B. S. Mittman, A. L. Siu, "Changing Provider Behavior: Applying Research on Outcomes and Effectiveness in Health Care," *Improving Health Policy and Management* (1992): 195–224; L. Kaegi, "Using Guidelines to Change Clinical Behavior: Dissemination through Area Health Education Centers and Geriatric Education Centers," *Quality Review Bulletin* 19, no. 5 (1993): 165–9; M. Van Amringe, T. E. Shannon, "Awareness, Assimilation, and Adoption: The Challenge of Effective Dissemination and the First AHCPR-Sponsored Guidelines," *Quality Review Bulletin* 18, no. 12 (1992): 397–404.

4. J. Grimshaw, I. Russell, "Effect of Clinical Guidelines on Medical Practice: A Systematic Review of Rigorous Evaluations," *Lancet* 342 (1993): 1317–22.

5. D. M. Cline et al., "Physician Compliance with Advanced Cardiac Life Support Guidelines," *Annals of Emergency Medicine* 25 (1995): 52–7.

6. L. M. Lewis, K. J. Welch, B. E. Ruof, "Failure of a Chest Pain Clinical Policy to Modify a Physician Evaluation and Management," *Annals of Emergency Medicine*

25 (1995): 9–14; R. Brook, "Implementing Practice Guidelines," *Lancet* 346 (1995): 132.

7. V. Fuchs, A. Garber, "The New Technology Assessment," *NEJM* 323, no. 10 (1990): 673–7; A. Linton, D. Naylor, "Organized Medicine and the Assessment of Technology: Lessons from Ontario," *NEJM* 323, no. 20 (1990): 1463–7.

8. S. R. Tunis et al., "Internists' Attitudes about Clinical Practice Guidelines," *Annals of Internal Medicine* 120, no. 11 (1994): 956–63.

9. U.S. Congress, Office of Technology Assessment, *Identifying Health Technologies That Work: Searching for Evidence* (Washington, D.C.: U.S. Congress, Office of Technology Assessment, September 1994).

10. The GUSTO Investigators, "An International Randomized Trial Comparing Four Thrombolytic Strategies for Acute Myocardial Infarction," *NEJM* 329, no. 10 (1993): 673–82.

11. S. E. Stool et al., "Otitis Media with Effusion in Young Children," *Clinical Practice Guidelines* 12, 1994. Agency for Health Care Policy and Research, Public Health Services, U.S. Department of Health and Human Services, Rockville, Md., AHCPR Publication No. 94-0622.

12. L. Culpepper, J. Sisk, "The Development of Practice Guidelines: A Case Study of Otitis Media with Effusion," this volume.

13. M. J. Field, K. N. Lohr, eds., *Clinical Practice Guidelines: Directions for a New Program,* Institute of Medicine (Washington, D.C.: National Academy Press, 1990); *A Guide to Establishing Programs for Assessing Outcomes in Clinical Settings,* Joint Commission on Accreditation of Healthcare Organizations (Oakbrook Terrace, Ill. 1994).

14. H. E. Whyte et al., "Extreme Immaturity: Outcome of 568 Pregnancies of 23–26 Weeks' Gestation," *Obstetrics and Gynecology,* no. 1 (1993): 81.

15. M. G. Allen et al., "The Limit of Viability—Neonatal Outcome of Infants Born at 22 to 25 Weeks' Gestation," *NEJM* 329, no. 22 (1993): 1597–1601.

16. R. M. Veatch, "Values in Routine Medical Decisions and the Concept of 'Medical Indications,'" in *The Patient-Physician Relation: The Patient as Partner, Part 2* (Bloomington, Ind.: Indiana University Press, 1991), pp. 47–62; R. M. Veatch, "Technology Assessment: Inevitability a Value Judgment," this volume.

17. D. Grady et al., "Hormone Therapy to Prevent Disease and Prolong Life in Postmenopausal Women," *Annals of Internal Medicine* 117, no. 12 (1992): 1016–37; "American College of Physicians, Guidelines for Counseling Postmenopausal Women about Preventative Hormone Therapy," *Annals of Internal Medicine* 117, no. 12 (1992): 1038–41; S. E. Bell, "Technology Assessment, Outcomes Data, and Social Context: The Case of Hormone Therapy," this volume.

18. S. E. Kelly, B. A. Koenig, "'Rescue' Technologies following High-Dose Chemotherapy for Breast Cancer: How Social Context Shapes the Assessment of Innovative, Aggressive, and Lifesaving Medical Technologies," this volume.

19. K. M. Taylor, "Physicians and the Disclosure of Information," in *Biomedicine Examined.* M. Lock and E. Gordon, eds. (Dordrecht: Kluwer Publishers, 1988), pp. 441–63.

20. A. Strauss et al., *Psychiatric Ideology and Institutions* (New York: Free Press).

21. T. W. Hu et al., "The Impact of California Proposition 99, a Major Anti-Smoking Law, on Cigarette Consumption," *Journal of Public Health Policy* 15, no. 1 (Spring 1994): 26–36. "The Tobacco Industry, State Politics, and Tobacco Education in California," *American Journal of Public Health* 83, no. 9 (September 1993): 1214–21.

22. T. J. Glynn, "Methods of Smoking Cessation—Finally, Some Answers," *JAMA* 263, no. 20 (May 23/30, 1990): 2795–6; M. Manley et al., "Clinical Interventions in Tobacco Control: A National Cancer Institute Training Program for Physicians," *JAMA* 266, no. 22 (December 11, 1991): 3172–3.

23. H. Beebe et al., "Assessing Risk Associated with Carotid Endarterectomy: A Statement for Health Professionals by an Ad Hoc Committee on Carotid Surgery Standards of the Stroke Council, American Heart Association" *Circulation* 79, no. 2 (1989): 472–3. C. M. Winslow et al., "The Appropriateness of Cartoid Endarterectomy," *NEJM* 318, no. 12 (1988): 721–7.

24. "Screening for High Blood Cholesterol," Guide to Clinical Preventive Services: An Assessment of the Effectiveness of 169 Interventions. Report of the U.S. Preventive Services Task Force (Baltimore, Md.: Williams & Wilkins) 1989: 11–22.

25. A. L. Hyams et al., "Practice Guidelines and Malpractice Litigation: A Two-Way Street," *Annals of Internal Medicine* 122 (1995): 450–5.

26. A. J. Rosoff, "The Role of Clinical Practice Guidelines in Health Care Reform," *Health Matrix* 5 (1995): 369–96; J. D. Ayres, "The Use and Abuse of Medical Practice Guidelines," *The Journal of Legal Medicine* 15 (1994): 421–43.

Ruth S. Hanft

Health Technology Assessment in the 1990s

Introduction and History

"Outcomes" and "effectiveness" have become the bywords of 1990s efforts, by public and private sectors, to increase efficiency in the delivery of health care. While the words "outcomes" and "effectiveness" may be new, they are a subset of the broader concept of "technology assessment," an old and still evolving science and art. In a sense, technology assessment has been with us since the inception of medical care; the trial and error of the physician who tests applied scientific knowledge could be considered a technology assessment. What characterizes more recent efforts in the systematic clinical assessment of health care technology is the analysis of social, economic, and ethical consequences of its use and the translating of findings into "best" practice at the provider/patient level.

There are numerous barriers to achieving the expected goals of technology assessment, including (but not exclusively) methodological questions in medicine and economics, the rapidity of scientific and technological change, and the failure by physicians and consumers to adopt findings. The discussion that follows will provide a brief history of health technology assessment in the United States. This includes the role of the public and private sectors in legitimizing this approach to health policy analysis, and the emergence of technology assessment as an issue in health care reform.

Technology Assessment before the 1970s

Technology assessment has long been a fundamental practice of the healing profession: observation, trial, and error by individual physicians. As the science of medicine evolved, formalized testing methods, such as case studies, series studies, clinical trials, and randomized-controlled trials, evolved. These methods and newer statistical methods, such as meta-analysis, are designed to provide physicians, patients, and policy makers with information on the probability that the drug, device, or procedure is safe and works, i.e., improves the patient's condition, saves lives, reduces disability, or improves the quality of life.

With changes in medical education in the early 1900s and the move toward a stronger scientific component to medical education and practice came the institutionalization of more systematic attention to what new scientific breakthroughs ought to be adopted. Formalized assessments of safety and efficacy began in the United States with food and drug legislation in 1923. The creation of the National Institutes of Health (NIH) in 1931 and the subsequent explosion of federal biomedical-research funding after World War II resulted in large-scale, decades-long clinical trials of new treatments for prevalent illnesses. Many of these trials were performed in the private sector and consisted of the testing of pharmaceuticals, a step required for the FDA preapproval process of new drugs. NIH in particular, however, also funded broad longitudinal trials, notably the Framingham trials.

Developments in the 1970s

The major health care issue in the 1970s was defined as escalating costs, particularly under the Medicare program. Congress, private payers, and economists sought to identify the causes of, and find acceptable solutions to, this health care inflation. One belief enjoying good currency was that technological advances played a major role in health care inflation. "There is an emerging consensus that many technologies have been widely adopted into medical practice in the face of disturbingly scanty information about their health benefits, clinical risks, cost effectiveness and social side effects."[1]

Even before the 1978 congressional hearings just quoted, a number of activities related to technology assessment and the relationship of technology to health care costs were taking place.

- In 1972, Congress established the Office of Technology Assessment as an analytic arm of the Congress. Although its charge was the assessment of all kinds of technology, it early became active in health technology assessment.
- In 1972, Congress enacted amendments to the Social Security Act requiring prior approval of capital investment by providers before Medicare would reimburse for certain capital expenses.[2]
- The act provided also for experiments with professional-standards review organizations to enforce appropriate utilization of services—primarily in-hospital services—for Medicare beneficiaries.
- In 1974, Congress enacted the Comprehensive Health Planning Act, which included certificate-of-need processes for public review and approval of major capital and equipment investment by hospitals.

- In 1976, Congress enacted legislation requiring that medical devices be subject to premarket approval and postmarket surveillance by the FDA, just as drugs were.
- In 1976, the National Institutes of Health initiated consensus conferences, which synthesize information and bring the judgment of professionals and nonprofessionals to bear on technology assessment issues.
- A conference at Sun Valley in 1977, titled "Medical Technology: The Culprit behind Health Care Costs?" represented further speculation about technology's costs in the public and private sectors.[3]

An equally important force behind technology assessment was the use of the term "medical necessity" by purchasers of health care. During the 1970s, the Social Security Administration (SSA), which was the administering agency for Medicare, began to implement more actively the "medical necessity" clause of the original program legislation. Under the law, Medicare, like most private health insurance, could pay only for medically necessary services. Similarly, it was precluded from paying for experimental or investigational drugs or procedures. Until the 1970s the SSA had made ad hoc inquiries to the FDA or NIH regarding coverage of specific technologies. A small office was established in the Office of the Assistant Secretary for Health to coordinate responses to Medicare from the Public Health Service agencies as the number of inquiries increased during the early 1970s.

Technology assessment gained important public recognition in 1978 when Congress established the National Center for Health Care Technology (NCHCT) to advise Medicare on coverage, to set priorities for technology assessment of newly emerging technologies, to convene and conduct assessments, and to disseminate the findings of technology assessment. The life of the center was brief. In 1982 the Reagan administration did not request an appropriation for the center and it died, only to be reborn in 1989. The coverage-related functions were transferred to the Office of Health Technology Assessment in the National Center for Health Services Research.[4]

Private-Sector Responses

Both the American Medical Association (AMA) and the Health Industry Manufacturers Association were opposed to the creation and activities of the NCHCT. Their objections were based primarily on the regulatory potential of the findings of systematic technology assessment. The NCHCT had no regulatory authority; its basic charter was research, coordination, and dissemination.

The American Medical Association established its own technology assessment initiative. Others in the private sector, particularly employers and insurers, began to look to technology assessment for help in constraining costs. The most notable private effort of this period was Blue Cross's request that the American College of Physicians assess the value of the routine laboratory tests and chest X rays required by most hospitals prior to admission.

During the late 1970s and early 1980s, clinicians and health services researchers at universities and research centers such as the RAND Corporation and Dartmouth Medical School turned their attention to what has come to be called outcomes research, including studies of variation in patterns of medical practice. The compilation of large computerized databases of private and public health care claims facilitated analysis of clinical behavior and health care utilization. Specialty societies, most notably the American College of Physicians, undertook their own studies or conducted studies at the request of others.

At roughly the same time, other forms of technology assessment were being developed. Because traditional technology assessment can be an expensive undertaking—large-scale randomized clinical trials can cost millions of dollars and take several years to complete—a number of researchers have begun to apply new methodologies for the analysis of outcomes. Similarly, meta-analysis, a sophisticated statistical technique, is being used to combine findings of multiple clinical trials or other research studies. One notable such study is the ongoing analysis of effective care in pregnancy and childbirth.[5] Also, quality-of-life measures (QALY) were developed as a substitute for economic measures. The former measure effectiveness in life years or disability days saved to avoid some of the technical and ethical limitations of a purely economic approach. Cost-effectiveness studies, for example, have methodological limitations and must be used with care.

When the National Center for Health Care Technology was disbanded in 1982, other quasi-public efforts were made by the Institute of Medicine of the National Academy of Sciences to maintain a focus on technology assessment. In 1980, the Institute of Medicine had convened a conference "linking the clinical use of biomedical technologies and the collection of evaluative data." Subsequently, a study group was convened to address the strengths and weaknesses of technology assessment methods, the translation of technology assessment into clinical care, and the financing of technology assessment. This committee produced a major document that addressed these issues.[6] In 1986, the Institute of Medicine established the Council on Health Care Technology, which functioned until 1990.

The Return of the Public Sector

In 1983, a dramatic change—that provided an impetus for technology assessment—was made in the way the Medicare program paid hospitals. The new methodology, payment per hospitalization according to so-called Diagnosis Related Groups (DRGs), changed the financial incentives for hospitals from spending more per admission to spending less without compromising care. Hospitals began to seek efficiencies in their use of resources—technological and otherwise.

In 1989, the National Center for Health Services Research was dramatically expanded in function, funding, and name, becoming the Agency for Health Care Policy and Research (AHCPR) and taking on the sponsorship of outcomes research and practice guidelines. A major initiative was undertaken in patient outcomes research with the funding of university-based Patient Outcome Research Teams (PORT), which conduct large-scale studies of the effectiveness of specific medical technologies. In addition, AHCPR oversees the development of practice guidelines.[7]

Even with the reinstatement of a formal technology assessment agency with expanded functions (once the purview of the NCHCT), federal government activities in technology assessment remain fragmented and uncoordinated. The legal and regulatory functions of the FDA focus on the safety and efficacy of drugs and devices, with little attention to, or authority over, economic considerations. NIH continues to sponsor consensus conferences that produce little behavioral change in the practice community. NIH is still the major source of clinical trials other than those for drugs and devices. The Veterans Administration and the Department of Defense also engage in technology assessment activities in connection with their clinical responsibilities.

In summary, federal efforts in the health care technology field, except for the regulatory functions regarding safety and efficacy of drugs and devices, have been sporadic and uncoordinated, with little focus or assessment, including in outcomes research. The process continues to be ad hoc.

As will be discussed, with the rapid move toward managed care and health care delivery system reform, considerable activity has begun in the private sector. Notably, the large managed care organizations are developing practice protocols/guidelines, and the pharmaceutical industry is pursuing developments in pharmacoeconomics research.

Issues for Public Payers

Medicare and Medicaid, particularly the latter, have been faced with rapidly rising expenditures leading to congressional and state efforts to stem the rising budgets. Two trends in state efforts to restrain Medicaid expenditures have been partially dependent on the results of outcomes and other effectiveness research.

First, the Oregon Medicaid experiment presupposed a public philosophy that only effective medical technology should be provided to Medicaid recipients. The hypothesis was that if ineffective or marginally effective medical care and the inappropriate use of technology could be eliminated, more low-income people could be provided with health insurance using the saved resources. Through a wide public consultative process, procedures were ranked by their expected effectiveness in diagnosis, treatment, increasing life expectancy, and avoidance of disability. This was the first large-scale experiment in linking coverage of services to expected outcomes. The major limitation of the approach was the paucity of scientific and economic outcomes data. The process of determining what should and should not be covered relied largely on professional consensus.

States are also rapidly moving toward enrolling Medicaid patients into managed care organizations, paying for services on a capitated rather than per service basis. In the former type of delivery system, the payer relies on the managed care organization to determine what procedures, modalities, and sites of care are cost-effective. Little is currently known about how managed care organizations make coverage decisions and how, other than by denying payment, they transmit effectiveness information to the medical practitioners. Some use standardized protocols or guidelines developed by their own physicians. The basis for the protocols may or may not be actual outcomes/effectiveness research. More likely they are based on "best judgments."

There has been periodic discussion of Medicare (HCFA) assuming a stronger role in effectiveness research. The proposals in general suggest that for newly emerging, promising, experimental/investigational technologies, Medicare should provide coverage through selected providers, mainly academic health centers, to collect outcomes data to assess the effectiveness of the technology. Such a strategy could vastly expand the funding of outcomes research and might serve as an incentive to private insurers and managed-care organizations to participate in individual studies.

Medical Necessity

The failure to enact a national health reform program leaves us with the current highly decentralized system of private market decision making and the Medicare and Medicaid coverage policies. "Medical necessity," a vague concept, remains the dominant standard for coverage determinations but is in the eye of the beholder.

What evidence is needed to determine medical necessity? How about safety and efficacy, effectiveness, cost-effectiveness? What do these terms mean? Whose definitions should prevail, and what is our confidence in the methods used to make each of the determinations? Whose decision is it?

"Medically necessary" has never been explicitly defined. Does it vary with the purchaser of health care—such as insurers or employers—whose profits and competitive position may influence coverage of new, expensive technology or the use of less costly modalities of care, which may or may not be the most effective? With the HMO, driven by similar incentives? Or does the meaning of medical necessity depend on the physician, whose ethos is to advocate for the patient but who is also influenced by economic incentives? Is the meaning ever determined by the consumer, who usually does not have adequate technical information and frequently does not experience the full economic burden of the decision? It may even come down to the courts, as in the notable case of bone marrow transplants for advanced breast cancer. These often conflicting meanings demonstrate that "medically necessary" is an amorphous concept and inherently involves value judgments and cultural mores.

Medical Outcomes

A number of HMOs have begun to contract with organizations such as the RAND Corporation or the various specialty societies to assist them in making outcomes/technology assessment decisions. Except for the limited guidelines activities of the AHCPR, the efforts of insurers and HMOs are highly decentralized. The decisions of one group in one region may not be the same as that of another group in another region, raising questions of consumer access to certain technologies. Recently, however, Milliman and Robertson, a private firm, has been developing standardized guidelines that are being used by an increasing number of insurers. Medical groups have criticized these guidelines as rigid and as promoting "cookbook" medicine, based on averages and administered with little flexibility regarding individual patients.

It is impossible and impractical to list every drug, device, and procedure that will be covered under what circumstances in a benefit package or insurance policy, so the consumer must rely on trust and, potentially, litigation. Coverage entails many discrete decisions based on scope of care for an individual or population.

It can be anticipated that as insurers and HMOs begin to implement outcomes findings and guidelines and as consumers perceive that potentially beneficial technologies are not available, the courts will become active in determining how far providers and insurers can go in implementing the findings of outcomes research and guidelines. The state of the art of assessment and the heavy reliance on professional judgment may presage increasing litigation over coverage decisions.

A related issue that has been debated for many years is, When is a technology investigational/experimental and when has it passed that stage and is a generally accepted modality of care? The AZT experience and the controversies over new cancer treatments are examples of ongoing debates.

Here the issue involves questions of basic safety and sufficient experience to determine if the technology works at all, and for what proportion of cases.

Finally, the effectiveness debate frequently confuses what works in a large number of cases and what is appropriate to use in a specific case. The use of magnetic resonance imaging (MRI) is a clear example. It can show brain abnormalities in a noninvasive way, but should it be used for all symptoms of headache or every time those diagnosed with nonpreventable small strokes faint? Should ultrasound or fetal monitors be used routinely?

Resource Allocation

Nationally we have not come to grips with the growing portion of the GDP spent for health care and have been unwilling to engage in serious discussions of resource allocation among health care and other societal priorities at the macro level. Only the Oregon Medicaid experiment explicitly addressed these issues, and regrettably it had to make certain micro decisions without adequate outcomes information available.

In a disaggregated system of financing health care, macro decisions can only be effected for the specific enrolled population in a specific health insurance plan. Macro decisions become difficult to sustain if purchasers of health care—employers, consumers, and government—can shift among alternative plans or if court cases overturn guidelines. Ultimately, given the role of the courts in the United States, a decentralized system will preclude macro resource allocation.

Under the current system and for the foreseeable future, therefore, micro decision making will prevail under private financing systems with some macro decision making possible for beneficiaries of federal and state programs. The role of outcomes research therefore can be expected (with the limitations of court decisions) to be applicable only to single insurers/HMOs and to the Medicare program.

Goals for Outcomes Research

Proponents have enumerated a number of expectations and goals for outcomes research and their translation into practice guidelines.

- Outcomes research can reduce unnecessary use of procedures/modalities of care. It is assumed that outcomes research can determine what is unnecessary and that these determinations can be applied in individual cases. It also assumes that the research is value-free.
- Outcomes research can improve the quality of care. The problem here is the definition and measurement of quality and who defines quality.

- Outcomes research can reduce cost. Cost is probably the driving force for outcomes research, but outcomes research could produce either cost-reducing or cost-enhancing results. The theory behind the cost-reducing assumption is that there is inappropriate use of technology and use of ineffective technology. Outcomes research cannot address the efficiency in production of a specific technology, for example, what is the most resource-conserving method of performing coronary artery bypass surgery?
- Outcomes research can provide information for provider/patient decision making. This is perhaps the most feasible goal for outcomes research, assuming clarity and widespread diffusion of the findings.

Skeptics criticize outcomes research for methodological reasons and for the problems of values inherent in the research and in its use. Values, however, should not preclude either the research itself or its use if the values are explicit. Outcomes research findings are but one tool in a complex decision-making process.

Roles of the Provider, the Payer, the Consumer, and the Political Process

In nations with national health plans, the political process and/or the government payer are the major "decision makers" in resource allocation at the macro level. In democratic societies, the polity/consumer plays an important role in the political process. Day-to-day decision making, excluding major resource allocation decisions that have been made, rest with the provider-consumer relationship. The findings of outcomes research and technology assessment are used, to a greater or lesser extent, for resource allocation decisions on total dollars spent, capital investment including manpower, and gross allocation by age and medical condition. Micro decision making has not been fully described in the literature but is in part dependent on the cultural mores of the country. There are, for example, substantial differences in the use of life-extending technologies for the terminally ill from nation to nation.

Without this framework of national payment for health care and/or a highly regulated public/private system, the United States is left with a multiplicity of macro decision points as well as micro ones. The best potential for outcomes research, guidelines, and technology assessment is to provide information that multiple decision makers can rely on for decentralized decision making.

A market approach presupposes that "the market" can rationally allocate resources. While this is questionable in an economic sector that is in part a public good/social good, it is our current system. Technology assessment in a market economy is an information tool to be used by buyers and sellers in making decisions. The challenge is to develop adequate methodologies, sound analysis, and sophisticated diffusion to provide the multiple players with the opportunity to operate in the market.

Conclusions

Formalized technology assessment that goes beyond the safety and efficacy of drugs and devices is still in its early stages and highly decentralized among insurers, HMOs, specialty societies, government agencies, and research and health benefits organizations. Other nations make macro resource allocation decisions, usually through supply control, leaving individual patient decisions to physicians and consumers. The United States, because of its decentralized financing systems, is moving in the direction of more diffuse and micro decision making by payers, limiting decision making by consumers and providers. With the proclivity for use of the courts to redress perceived inequity, it can be expected that guidelines and the implementation of the findings of outcomes research will be increasingly challenged in the courts.

NOTES

1. U.S. Congress, House of Representatives, 95th Congress, 2nd Session Report #95-1190 by the Committee on Interstate and Foreign Commerce; Health Services Research, Statistics and Health Care Technology Act (Washington, DC: USGPO 1978).
2. Sec. 1122, Social Security Act.
3. "Medical Technology: The Culprit behind Health Care Costs?" Proceedings of the 1977 Sun Valley Forum on National Health.
4. R. A. Rettig, *Health Affairs* 12, no. 3 (1994); Seymour Perry, "The Brief Life of the National Center for Health Care Technology," *NEJM* 307 (1982): 1095–1100.
5. M. Enkin, M. Keirse, and I. Chalmers, *A Guide to Effective Care in Pregnancy and Childbirth* (Oxford: Oxford University Press, 1989).
6. U.S. Congress, Office of Technology Assessment, *Assessing Medical Technology* (Washington, D.C.: National Academy Press, 1985).
7. R. A. Rettig, "Medical Technology."

Paul J. Edelson

Clinical Practice Guidelines: A Historical Perspective on Their Origins and Significance

Practice guidelines originate in the phenomenon of practice pattern variations described by Wennberg and his associates in a continuing series of studies beginning in the mid-1970s.[1] These papers demonstrated substantial geographical variation in the aggregate use of physician[2] and hospital[3] services and in specific utilization rates of common surgical[4] and radiologic[5] procedures. Such variations, occurring over relatively small geographic areas, have now been documented for hospital services in several countries,[6] for children's hospitalizations,[7] and for rates of rehospitalization of elderly patients,[8] both by Wennberg's group and by others.[9] Although these authors[10] have argued that these variations neither reflect an intrinsic variation in the prevalence of specific conditions[11] nor are explained solely by differing patient preferences,[12] what they do represent is still a matter of considerable debate.[13] Nonetheless, there appears to be general agreement that such variations are a symptom of something seriously wrong with our medical system,[14] which should be addressed either for its own sake[15] or as a way of controlling medical-care costs.[16]

Such a thorough rejection of practice variations, however,[17] is far from the attitude that most American physicians have held about the nature of medical practice. As long as physicians have focused on the treatment of disease as "the great end of all our studies"—as the famous nineteenth-century American physician Austin Flint, Sr.,[18] expressed the preeminent significance of therapeutics for medical practice—it has been recognized that an essential characteristic of medical therapy, i.e., drugs, was that to be conscientious, it could not be routine. There were at least two reasons for this. First, because the expression of disease varied not only with the nature of the disease but also with the nature of the patient, the drugs used to treat the condition would reflect both the specific disease and the specific individual who was sick. And second, because all drugs had many different actions, the risks of what we might call the side effects of a drug in a given patient might vary with the patient's temperament and constitution. Thus, if one had two drugs with a similar action, say, two cathartics, from which to choose, and if one tended secondarily to be a stimulant while the second was not, one might prefer the first drug for an otherwise robust young man whose disease required a purgative, as he might be restored more promptly to his usual state of good health by its stimulant effects, while the second drug might be preferred for a frail elderly woman who might not tolerate excessive stimulation.

At the core of this perspective is the concept that care of the patient must be individualized. No two patients ever have exactly the same disorder, and therefore proper treatment must be based not only on the specific or, as Sydenham called them, the "constant" features of the patient's disease but also on a range of personal characteristics that distinguish one patient from another, and one patient's personal disorder[19] from another's. Such individual differences in disease implied a requirement for a similar individualization of therapy. As an editorialist for the *Boston Medical and Surgical Journal* put it in 1883, "No two instances of typhoid fever or of any other disease are precisely alike. No 'rule of thumb,' no recourse to a formula-book, will avail the treatment even of the typical disease."[20]

This was not to deny any systematic relationship between a patient's illness and its proper treatment but, rather, to insist that treatment could not be mechanically chosen without attention to a wide range of characteristics of which the physician would be aware as part of the patient's personal or family history or that would be recognized as the disease expressed itself in that particular patient. As Dunglinson put it in his popular manual for medical practitioners: "While it is allowed that formulae may often be employed with great advantage, yet they should not be prescribed with servile exactness; for it should never be forgotten that all medicines of any power have to be adapted to the requirements of the special case under treatment. It has been quaintly but truly observed, that a bundle of ready-made receipts in the hands of the routine practitioner is but a well-equipped quiver on the back of an unskillful archer."[21]

Therapeutically important characteristics have, at various times, included personal, hereditary, and familial factors, race, sex, age, social class, personal temperament, and other "constitutional proclivities."[22] But while the list of specific factors that are taken into account by the physician has varied over time, medicine's essential attitude was consistently that of commitment to the principle of "therapeutic specificity."[23] And this commitment to therapeutic individualization was seen as an essential component of the physician's professional identity.

As the historian John Harley Warner emphasizes in his superb study of American medical practice,[24] well into the nineteenth century the categorical use of specific therapies was widely considered the mark of the incompetent practitioner, if not of the medical quack. Not only distinguished authors of medical textbooks[25] but also ordinary medical practitioners were concerned about the dangers of mechanical therapeutics, as evidenced in this quotation from a letter written in 1822 by a Kentucky practitioner to his brother: "I do not wish to see you a mere *Blue Pill Peddlar* nor doctor who carries in his Pockets something that is *good for* this & that complaint."[26]

One of the chief criticisms of such medical sects as Thompsonianism and homeopathy was their "cookbook"-like approaches to therapeutics with specific recipes listed in their textbooks for each disease.[27] As a professor of orthodox medicine at the University of Michigan put it in 1855, the various elements that the principle of specificity required physicians to take into account when determining the proper treatment included: "Age of the Patient. The Sex . . . Constitution . . . The temperament. The disease going on in the organ. Idiosyncrasies, or personal peculiarities. Variation of the pulse. Habits of the patient. Tolerance of medicines. Climate. The prevailing epidemic influence. Race. Profession. Severity of the disease."[28]

Such a broad definition of factors influencing the expression of disease and therefore necessary to consider in selecting an appropriate therapy, while emphasizing the importance of the patient as an individual in the medical encounter, also opened the way to the intrusion of various social prejudices that denied the same potential for suffering or the same vulnerability to disease from one class to another. Pernick has extensively documented the class biases that retarded the use of anesthesia for Victorian soldiers and laborers, who were seen as being less susceptible to pain than members of the more "refined" levels of society,[29] while Savitt has described the ideology of "Southern" medicine and its categorical differentiation of diseases in black and white patients.[30] In some cases, as when it was used as an argument against laypeople's self-dosing, the ideology of individuality was used more to further the professional interests of physicians than to assure patients individualized care.[31]

The doctrine of individuality, however, also had other, more positive effects on patient care. By emphasizing the therapeutic importance of a continuing relationship between doctor and patient, it became a major support for the importance of the general physician in his response to the competition of medical specialization. According to many medical leaders,[32] it was precisely his greater access to a patient's individual and familial idiosyncracies that made the family physician better qualified than the specialist to treat most illnesses and assured the elder physician a competitive advantage against the new graduate.[33]

This traditional understanding of the individuality of patients and their diseases did not go completely unchallenged. Indeed, as early as the seventeenth century it was attacked by those favoring the concept of diseases as biologic species, rather than differing circumstances of one's physiologic balance. A tension between individuality and category is evident in the writings of Thomas Sydenham, the eighteenth-century physician who was called the "English Hippocrates" because of his efforts to systematize disease categories according to their characteristic signs and symptoms. He struggled with distinguishing between what he called "constant" and "adventitious" symptoms, arguing that diagnoses should be based only on the constant or categorical elements of an illness and not on its incidental or adventitious features.[34] Such an approach to diagnosis, based on what we would understand to be systematic objective criteria, would seem to represent a great advance in comparison with earlier and more indefinite diagnostic systems. But such approaches also carried with them serious consequences for the traditional therapeutic relationship between doctor and patient. As Reiser has noted, "Combining patients into categories (populations) [was a] major step in physicians' growing detachment from the unique traits of their patients . . . [and] reduced their empathic concerns."[35]

In other words, by introducing an objective system of diagnosis and characterizing patients' conditions strictly according to such a system, physicians were ignoring precisely those individual characteristics that the older medicine had required them to systematically define and respect. I would argue that it is this "growing detachment" from its patients that has been a principal, though highly contentious, theme of modern scientific medical practice and that the failure of medicine to appreciate the consequences of this new definition of the job of the doctor has undercut some of the technical successes that modern medicine has achieved.[36]

The tradition of individualized treatment was widely shared not only by physicians and other medical practitioners but also by the public in general. Studies of the social history of medical practice[37] make clear that therapeutic individualization was common in the eighteenth century and that tailoring therapeutic courses to the individual was routinely expected by patients and practiced by physicians. By the nineteenth century, however, with the growth of an increasingly materialistic general culture, physicians began to accept the concept of specific diseases and to redefine the therapeutic encounter as one in which drugs played a more central role, becoming, as the Porters put it, a "medium of exchange between physicians and patients."[38]

To some degree, it might be argued that the affective nexus that traditionally joined doctor and patient began to be supplanted by a "pharmaceutical" nexus symbolized by the prescription. But such a concrete, material link could not fully replace the elaborately defined cultural relationship of doctor and patient promoted by the doctrine of individualization. Instead, it tended to reduce the significance of the doctor-patient relationship to a more unidimensional commercial transaction, stripped of much of its positive social and symbolic meaning for both physician and patient. Such a diminished relationship may be less emotionally satisfactory to the participants, less able to recruit the patient's sympathies in carrying out his therapeutic regimen, and even less effective in helping to restore the patient's health.

The poverty of such an approach is emphasized in Tanenbaum's description of the varieties of physician accountability, in which it is clear that full professional accountability emerges only under conditions in which the physician is personally invested in the outcome of her care and where, rather than acting out a radically new role as administrative functionary in a world highly reminiscent of Weber's picture of the modern impersonal bureaucracy, the physician must, and is expected to, contribute some of her own personal energies to the relationship. Indeed, it is the process of individualizing therapy for a given patient, based in part on the patient's specific circumstances and in part on what Tanenbaum[39] refers to as the physician's "personal knowledge," that is the channel for expressing and sustaining such an investment. Such personal investment in the care of patients is, of course, in keeping with the highest traditions of humane medicine in our culture.

Such a commitment to the individuality of the patient need not be in conflict with the use of clinical norms or population-based data in assessing certain aspects of a physician's practice. But it would appear to be incompatible with some of the current practices of patient-by-patient assessment of medical care in which population-based practice data are applied to individual medical encounters—as if the overall expectation of 50 percent "heads" required that an honest coin come up "heads" every other time it is flipped. And most important, it carries with it the potential for further depleting the physician-patient relationship of that core recognition of each participant as an individual that both patients and physicians expect and that, in the Western tradition, the best medical care requires. While I would agree with Berwick[40] that the practice of "total quality management," as one of the more recent incarnations of administratively structured medical practice has been named, has the potential for "redefining doctoring," I would be cautious not to assume that such redefinition will not harm some of the qualities we most value in the doctor-patient relationship. As shrewd observers of the current efforts to overhaul medical care have noted, the debates over techniques to standardize clinical practices is a conflict of "policy choices, not scientific imperatives."[41]

Protocol-based uniformity is subject to the failure to recognize the "complexity of health care,"[42] just as it is characteristic of current political debate that complexity is one of the first things to be discarded. In such an environment it would seem prudent to tailor our remedy to both the strengths and the weaknesses of the system.

NOTES

1. J. E. Wennberg, A. Gittlesohn, and D. Soule, "Health Care Delivery in Maine I: Patterns of Use of Common Surgical Procedures," *J Maine Med Assoc* 66 (1975): 123–30.

2. W. P. Welch, "Geographic Variation in Expenditures for Physicians' Services in the United States," *NEJM* 328 (1993): 621–7.

3. J. E. Wennberg et al., "Hospital Use and Mortality among Medicare Beneficiaries in Boston and New Haven," *NEJM* 321 (1989): 1168–73.

4. J. E. Wennberg et al., "An Assessment of Prostatectomy for Benign Urinary Tract Obstruction: Geographic Variations and the Evaluation of Medical Care Outcomes," *JAMA* 259 (1988): 3027–30.

5. J. McNeill, D. Tihansky, and J. E. Wennberg, "Use of Medical Radiographs: Extent of Variation and Associated Active Bone Marrow Doses," *Radiology* 156 (1985): 51–6.

6. McPherson et al., "Small-Area Variations in the Use of Common Surgical Procedures: An International Comparison of New England, England, and Norway," *NEJM* 307 (1982): 1310–4.

7. Perrin et al., "Variations in Rates of Hospitalization of Children in Three Urban Communities," *NEJM* 320 (1989): 1183–7.

8. E. S. Fisher, "Hospital Readmission Rates for Cohorts of Medicare Beneficiaries in Boston and New Haven," *NEJM* 331 (1994): 989–95.

9. Chassin et al., "Variations in the Use of Medical and Surgical Services by the Medicare Population," *NEJM* 314 (1986): 285–90; J. Holahan, R. A. Berenson, and P. G. Kachavos, "Area Variations in Selected Medicare Procedures," *Health Affairs* 9 (1990): 166–75.

10. M. R. Chassin et al., "Does Inappropriate Use Explain Geographic Variations in the Use of Health Care Services? A Study of Three Procedures," *JAMA* 258 (1987): 2533–7.

11. J. E. Wennberg, "Population Illness Rates Do Not Explain Population Hospitalization Rates: A Comment on Mark Blumberg's Thesis That Morbidity Adjusters Are Needed to Interpret Small Area Variations," *Medical Care* 25 (1987): 354–9.

12. J. E. Wennberg and F. J. Fowler, Jr., "A Test of the Consumer Contribution to Small Area Variations in Health Care Delivery," *J Maine Med Assoc* 68 (1977): 275–9.

13. N. P. Roos and L. L. Roos, "Surgical Rate Variations: Do They Reflect the Health or Socioeconomic Characteristics of the Population?" *Medical Care* 20 (1982): 945–58.

14. J. E. Wennberg, "Unwanted Variations in the Rules of Practice," *JAMA* 265 (1991): 1306–7.

15. J. E. Wennberg, "Dealing with Medical Practice Variations: A Proposal for Action," *Health Affairs* 3 (1984): 6–32.

16. J. B. Rice, "Volume Performance Standards: Can They Control Growth in Medicare Services?" *Milbank Quarterly* 68 (1990): 295–319.

17. The presumption that both rates can't be right—a presumption that historically many American physicians would have considerable difficulty accepting—is reflected in the title of Wennberg's editorial commenting on another study demonstrating "small-area practice pattern variations." See J. E. Wennberg, "Which Rate Is Right?" *NEJM* 314 (1986): 310–1.

18. A. Flint, *A Treatise on the Principles and Practice of Medicine* (Philadelphia, 1867), p. 114.

19. It might be noted that this distinction between the features of the categorical disease and its appearance in an individual patient is in some ways echoed by recent differentiation in the usage of the terms "disease" and "illness." See, for example, A. Kleinman, *The Illness Narratives: Suffering, Healing, and the Human Condition* (New York: Basic Books, 1988).

20. "Routine Practice" (editorial), *Boston Med Surg J* 108 (1883): 43, cited in C.E. Rosenberg, "The Therapeutic Revolution: Medicine, Meaning, and Social Change in Nineteenth-Century America," in *The Therapeutic Revolution: Essays in the Social History of American Medicine,* M. J. Vogel and C. E. Rosenberg, eds. (Philadelphia: University of Pennsylvania Press, 1979), p. 19.

21. Dunglinson, *The Practitioner's Ready Reference Book* (Philadelphia, 1883), p. 75. Note that where Dunglinson uses the term "formulae" he is referring to the typical prescription formulations used in practice at the time. He uses the term "receipts" (or recipes) in the same way.

22. Lee, "How Far Does a Scientific Therapy Depend upon Materia Medica?" *JAMA* 31 (1898): 827, cited in Rosenberg, "The Therapeutic Revolution," p. 19.

23. H. Warner, *The Therapeutic Perspective: Medical Knowledge, Practice, and Professional Identity in America, 1820–1885* (Cambridge: Harvard University Press, 1984). See especially pp. 146 ff.

24. Warner, *The Therapeutic Perspective.*

25. See, for example, the widely used textbooks by R. Dunglinson, *Materia Medica and Therapeutics,* 8th ed. (New York, 1894).

26. Warner, *The Therapeutic Perspective*, p. 60, note 9.

27. Warner, *The Therapeutic Perspective*, p. 60, note 8.

28. Warner, *The Therapeutic Perspective,* pp. 58–9, note 1.

29. Pernick, *A Calculus of Suffering: Pain, Professionalism, and Anesthesia in Nineteenth-Century America* (New York: Columbia University Press, 1985).

30. Savitt, *Medicine and Slavery: The Diseases and Health Care of Blacks in Antebellum Virginia* (Ann Arbor, Michigan: Books on Demand, 1978).

31. H. Warner, "The Use of Southern Medical Distinctiveness: Medical Knowledge and Practice in the Old South," in *Science and Medicine in the Old South,* R. L. Numbers and T. L. Savitt, eds. (Baton Rouge, Louisiana State University Press, 1989), pp. 179–205.

32. See, for example, W. Osler, "Remarks on Specialism," *Arch Peds* 9 (1892): 481, cited in H. Cushing, *The Life of Sir William Osler, Bt.* (Oxford, Clarendon Press, 1925), vol. 1, p. 360.

33. As the dean of the Harvard Medical School, Oliver Wendell Holmes, put it: "The young man knows the rules, but the old man knows the exceptions. The young man knows his patient, but the old man knows also his patient's family, dead and alive, up and down for generations," From "The Young Practitioner," In *Medical Essays, 1842–1882* (Boston, 1882), p. 377.

34. T. Sydenham, "Medical Observations Concerning the History and Cure of Acute Diseases," In *The Works of Thomas Sydenham, MD*, vol. 1, T. G. Lathan, trans. (London, 1850).

35. S. J. Reiser, "Science, Pedagogy, and the Transformation of Empathy in Medicine," in *Empathy and the Practice of Medicine: Beyond the Pill and the Scalpel*, H. Spiro, M. G. McCurnen, E. Peschel, and D. St. James, eds. (New Haven: Yale University Press, 1993), p. 124.

36. C. Barnett and D. Rabin, "Collaborative Study by Physicians and Anthropologists: Congenital Hip Disease," In *The People's Health*, J. Adair and K. W. Deuschle, eds. (New Mexico: University of New Mexico Press, 1970). This is a fascinating account of how modern Western physicians developed an aggressive medical plan to treat congenital hip dislocation, a common condition in Navajo babies, only to have their therapy rejected by mothers who did not feel the need to "treat" a condition that was not a disability in Navajo life. Note here, again, that by the lights of current usage, the authors appear to have made the right choice in using *disease* rather than *illness* in discussing the condition of congenital hip dislocation among the Navajo.

37. A leading example of such modern studies is D. Porter and R. Porter, *Patient's Progress: Doctors and Doctoring in Eighteenth-Century England* (Stanford; Stanford University Press, 1898). See for example, p. 161.

38. Porter and Porter, *Patient's Progress*, p. 172.

39. S. J. Tanenbaum, "What Physicians Know," *NEJM* 329 (1993): 1268–70.

40. D. M. Berwick, "TQM: Redefining Doctoring," *Internist* 34 (1993): 8–10.

41. M. Werner, "Can Medical Decisions Be Standardized? Should They Be?" *Clin Chem* 39 (1993): 1361–8.

42. M. McKee and A. Clarke, "Guidelines, Enthusiasms, Uncertainty, and the Limits of Purchasing," *BMJ* 320 (1995): 101–4.

PART II: Outcomes Data

JUDITH WILSON ROSS
Practice Guidelines: Texts in Search of Authority

LARRY CULPEPPER AND JANE SISK
The Development of Practice Guidelines: A Case Study of Otitis Media with Effusion

GERT JAN VAN DER WILT AND PIETER F. DE VRIES ROBBÉ
The Quest for the Trial to End All Trials: The Case of Technology Assessment and Management of Glue Ear

DONALD J. MURPHY
Guideline Glitches: Measurements, Money, and Malpractice

SUSAN E. BELL
Technology Assessment, Outcomes Data, and Social Context: The Case of Hormone Therapy

SUSAN E. KELLEY AND BARBARA A. KOENIG
"Rescue" Technologies following High-Dose Chemotherapy for Breast Cancer: How Social Context Shapes the Assessment of Innovative, Aggressive, and Lifesaving Medical Technologies

DICK WILLEMS
Outcomes, Guidelines, and Implementation in France, the Netherlands, and Great Britain

Judith Wilson Ross

Practice Guidelines: Texts in Search of Authority

Introduction

Practice guidelines are both a well-established medical practice and a new phenomenon. Although general rules about how to proceed when practicing the art of medicine have a long history, the rigorous formulation of such guidelines is something new. One hope for guidelines, in the face of extensive practice variations observed twenty years ago by Wennberg, was that medical practice could be made more rational and scientific. A more scientific medicine would also produce a more professional medicine. Patients could be more confident that similar illnesses would be diagnosed and treated similarly, regardless of where they received their treatment. Guidelines have also been seen as a way of reducing health care costs because reliance on these more scientific guidelines would eliminate what was thought to be extensive inappropriate treatment provision.

All three of these hopes may prove unfounded. Research data are often inadequate or nonexistent, and thus cannot be used to create a scientific medical practice. Even among those treatments and conditions that have been well studied, research methodologies are flawed or inconsistent; randomized clinical trials—the gold standard—are hard to find. Thus, uncertainty remains. The hope that a more rational medicine would bolster professional values has also been problematic, as physicians have been reluctant to listen to others' views in the face of a history that treated them as individual entrepreneurs and (near) final arbiters of what treatment should be provided to patients. Last, the hope that guidelines would reduce costs by eliminating inappropriate treatment has had to be reconsidered. The practice variations literature has not led to the expected conclusion that variations result from overuse. Indeed, the source of variation remains somewhat mysterious.[1] It is clear, however, that implementation of guidelines might result in increased treatment and associated costs because it would remedy extensive underuse of some treatment, in addition to overuse.

Although the initial hopes that accompanied guidelines seem problematic, guidelines continue to be produced at a rapid rate. Those who produce them hope to change physician practice. The most direct way to alter practice would be to tie guidelines to reimbursement, a practice increasingly used by insurers. But those within the medical profession who see practice guidelines primarily as a way of improving medical care rather than reducing costs have not usually connected compliance to reimbursement, not least because it is a heavy-handed and punitive method of ensuring behaviors. Further, guidelines created to control costs might be perceived as being based upon arbitrary or profit-maximizing judgments rather than upon professionally responsible judgments intended to improve the quality of care for vulnerable patients. Good science would be the preferred basis for effective guidelines.

Those involved in guidelines development are fairly consistent in talking about guidelines as scientific and as rational approaches to treatment decisions. For example, Phelps describes guidelines development as one way of "developing a stronger scientific basis for medical decision making."[2] Fletcher and Fletcher, editors of *Annals of Internal Medicine,* say that "the development of practice guidelines results *naturally* from the application of scientific methods to the practice of medicine"[3] (italics added). This kind of language suggests— at least to the casual reader—that the guidelines' task is to say whether particular treatments actually worked and, if they did, under what circumstances they worked and thus should be offered to patients. Eddy, who describes practice guidelines as "generic decisions," also reinforces the idea that these are some kind of abstract truths in the form of rules.[4] This sense of guidelines as rules presumably led Brook to describe practice guidelines as telling physicians "what to do."[5] Yet there were disputes about what constituted "science." Some believed guidelines should be based solely on outcomes data derived from randomized clinical trials. Others argued that experts in the field who had at their fingertips the best available research should be able to make good judgments about what the rules should be. Richard Peto, who supported outcomes research, complained in an interview that "opinions do not define the word 'appropriate'" and went on to describe the use of expert panels as work that is "utterly self-referential. All it tells you is that the group of doctors you cobbled together recommends something."[6] Brook in reply claimed, according to the interviewer, that "expert opinion must count as data."[7]

Brooks's claim is important because research data—what Peto wants to use—are usually absent. In this absence, a central question arises about the authority of guidelines. If guidelines are to change practice, they must be authoritative; but if they are derived from opinion (even expert or informed

Practice Guidelines: Texts in Search of Authority   43

opinion) in the absence of good outcomes data (or if the outcomes are limited only to such parameters as morbidity and mortality), how can they be understood as authoritative? Two choices present themselves if guidelines are to be authoritative: they must depend either on substantive authority (i.e., they must emphasize their science) or on process authority (i.e., they must emphasize their process).

By looking at guidelines themselves, how they are structured, the language they use, and the aspects they emphasize, we can understand something about how guidelines developers do or don't use these methods to assert authority. For the purposes of this chapter, four different guidelines representing attempts by important professional groups to rationalize medical practice were analyzed: the National Institutes of Health (NIH) Consensus Conference ovarian cancer screening and treatment guideline, the American College of Physicians (ACP) hormone replacement guideline, the RAND Corporation cataract surgery guideline, and the Agency for Health Care Policy and Research (AHCPR) otitis media with effusion guideline. The four show large differences in their emphasis on substantive and procedural authority.

In order to understand something about the different ways that guidelines can express authoritativeness, eight areas were assessed:

Substantive Authority:

1) Is there a formal method by which the panel addresses the research literature?
2) Is the connection between data and recommendations made clear?
3) Does the methodology lead to quantifiable results at any point?

Procedural Authority:

4) Is there a defined method to create recommendations after substantive issues have been addressed?
5) Is the method of selecting panelists specified, and is the selection inclusive?
6) Is the process open to the public?
7) Are patient preferences and values accounted for in the process?
8) Are the guidelines broadly disseminated?

Substantive questions are important with respect to authoritativeness just because this is a question about scientific authority. Even though data are inadequate in most instances to ground recommendations solidly, demonstrating knowledge about, and methods of, interpreting data will permit such science as does exist to lend authority to the project. Thus, if guidelines are

44 Part II: Outcomes Data

to be perceived as authoritative on the basis of their science, one might expect that guideline creators would clearly describe the method by which research data are gathered and interpreted, would make the connection between the data and the recommendations as transparent as possible, and would develop some quantified material when creating recommendations because quantified material makes decision making appear more reliable and accurate. Process authority, on the other hand, would be more likely to emphasize issues of fairness. Given the uncertain nature of the science, guidelines would appear more authoritative if they could demonstrate a clear and replicable process method, appropriate expertise and inclusiveness in selecting those who produce the guidelines, a public process, some attempt to incorporate patient preferences and values, and a commitment to broad dissemination of the results.

Of the four guidelines under consideration, the ACP guideline depends more on substantive claims for authority, while the AHCPR and NIH guidelines show more process authority claims. The RAND guideline lies somewhere in between because it has a very detailed and quantified process methodology but a near complete disjunction between the substantive and process questions.

NIH Consensus Conference Guideline on Ovarian Cancer: Screening, Treatment, and Follow-up[8]

Description of the Consensus Conference

The fourteen-member NIH panel convenes like a jury (by its own description) and, with a public audience, listens to invited individuals provide expert testimony on specific aspects of the question. An extensive bibliography as well as some abstracts drawn from that bibliography are provided for the panel. The testimony is expected to place outcomes research in the proper perspective for the consensus panel. After hearing this evidence, the panel then meets in private and draws its conclusions from this testimony, creating a draft consensus statement. This draft is provided to the expert "witnesses" and to the public audience. After receipt of comments, the consensus statement is then revised and subsequently published in the medical literature.

Literature Review

The text of the NIH Conference states that abstracts and bibliographies are circulated to panelists, and bibliographies to the audience. The literature search is not otherwise explained. The expert witnesses provide an additional aspect of the literature review because they are asked to "testify" to help the panelists weigh the scientific evidence. Only one person is invited to address each topic that the panelists (presumably) wish addressed. No explanation is provided about how either the topics or the experts are chosen. Furthermore, although the experts testify in public session, no mention is made of published testimony. As a result, those who are to use the guideline have no way of understanding what issues were discussed or how those issues were presented with respect to the research data.

Connection between Data and Recommendations

As noted above, the guideline presents conclusions drawn from outcomes data, but there is no evaluation of the data presented in or with the guidelines. The panel's recommendations are, in a number of instances, loosely connected to or fully disconnected from the conclusions that the panel says may be drawn from the research. For example, the panel concludes that "[t]here are no data demonstrating that screening these high-risk women [with hereditary ovarian cancer syndrome] reduces their mortality from ovarian cancer." Nonetheless "at least annual rectovaginal pelvic examination, CA-125 determinations, and TVS are recommended in these women." Using "and" suggests that, despite the absence of data demonstrating reduced mortality, not one but all three screening mechanisms are to be recommended annually.

Finally, the panel's recommendations are frequently offered on the basis of unspecified judgments of confidence (e.g., "sufficiently high" or "sufficiently low" with no explanation of what constitutes a sufficiency). This further undermines claims to scientific legitimacy that are rhetorically made in the guideline text. (For example, from the abstract: "The panel, answering predefined consensus questions, developed their conclusions based on the scientific evidence presented in open forum and the scientific literature.")

Quantified Conclusions

Nothing is quantified in the NIH Consensus Conference guideline.

Formal Method

The NIH Consensus Conference emphasizes process, not methodology, but even then makes little attempt (beyond rhetoric) to explain its method. It describes itself as a "jury" hearing evidence in a public setting. There is no discussion of what constitutes evidence or how the jury is to consider the evidence. This is a strange jury process: one without a judge, without opposing attorneys to ensure that all sides are heard, and with expert witnesses whose qualifications are undemonstrated. By using the jury image, however, the Consensus Conference claims for its final recommendations more authority than it could otherwise claim.

Inclusiveness and Selection Procedures

Involving various members of the public who are not physicians could be an important, legitimating aspect of the guideline. This is understandable in terms of current rhetoric about "inclusion" and "empowerment" of those who are understood to be without power (patients generally, but particularly women patients in the case of this guideline). The abstract of this guideline accurately describes the fourteen-member panel as one that "represented" specialty physicians and statisticians. The text, however, describes it as a "panel with public and patient representation." Members of the 500-person audience presumably included at least some lay public and patients, but the expert witnesses did not. In any case, the witnesses and the audience are not "the panel." The panel included only one nonphysician, nonscientist who could reasonably be referred to as a representative of the "public and patient." She was an attorney, listed as the volunteer director of a pediatric cancer foundation. The phrase "public and patient representation," however, suggests more than one person (although it is not clear in what sense the "public" and the "patient" constitute different groups). In this area, the guideline asserts a claim to authority through patient and public inclusiveness, but there is not much behind the claim.

Although there is no agreement about which professionals should participate in guideline construction or what balance should be struck between various dualities when appointing panelists (e.g., between community versus academic physicians; researchers versus clinicians; specialists versus primary care physicians), some guidelines present "credentials" on these issues. The NIH document makes no claims beyond listing the names and affiliations of the panelists and the names and subjects of expertise of the expert witnesses. This listing reveals that the panel physicians are all specialists, and academic physicians outnumber private practice physicians by five to one.

The guideline text itself is attentive to the issue of panelist representation. Abstract, text, and notes use the following phrases to describe the panelists: "independent," "nonfederal," and "nonadvocate." These terms are apparently intended to allay fears about special interests or fears that physicians will be influenced in decision making by their own economic interests. If guideline recommendations come from those who are "independent," "nonfederal," and "nonadvocate," the implication is that the judgments will not be tainted by self-interest or by special pleading. Yet we are not told what it is that the panelists are independent of, what it is that they do not advocate. Eleven of the fourteen are affiliated with universities[9] and are probably at least occasional recipients of federal research funds. If not federal employees, they are in most cases state employees because their appointments are in state universities.

By contrast, the expert witnesses are listed (with their topics of expertise) in the consensus publication, but their affiliations are not listed. Perhaps this means that NIH cannot vouch for their independence or nonadvocacy or nonfederalness, but the more probable implication is that concerns about representativeness and independence are relevant only for the panelists. Still, because the panelists appear to rely on expert witnesses to evaluate the research, the witnesses' independence is also an issue. The problem for NIH, however, is that those who have the most expertise and thus are most likely to be selected as witnesses are also more likely to be advocates for the procedure/treatment in question.

Public Nature of Process

The NIH guideline also emphasizes (in the published abstract) that the panel "developed their conclusions based on the scientific evidence presented in open forum and the scientific literature," a twofold authority claim. The implication is that "doctors working in secret" would not be tolerable. But what the NIH consensus conference panel actually does is spend one and a half days in an open-forum discussion and the next one and a half days making its decision behind closed doors, issuing the final revision "within a few weeks after the conference," when the experts and the audience are no longer around. Although this is, pragmatically, a sensible way to manage the problem of getting a group of people to produce a written consensus statement, the text emphasizes—and thereby claims credit for—the openness of the process. This claim for authority is not fully justified, of course.

Breadth of Dissemination

Although one might think that "the main objective of . . . guidelines is to help physicians in their daily practice,"[10] they are more often described in terms of physician and patient decision making. By promoting dissemination to patients as well as physicians, the guideline could be more widely known and could more likely result in conversations between physicians and patients so that patient decision making could be enhanced.

The NIH guideline states that its purpose is to make judgments about current research so that "healthcare providers will have all these data available to them and so that all women can benefit from this information" (abstract, p. 491). Yet the NIH consensus guideline is addressed only to practitioners and is published only in medical journals. Although the text states that it is intended to benefit women and the notes say it is "to be useful . . . to the public," this use is apparently to be mediated solely through physicians.

Patient Preferences

Roche and Durieux[11] suggest that patient preference is an integral part of the guideline because appropriate medical care is defined in terms of benefits outweighing risks. Because patients and clinicians may weigh both risks and benefits differently, only patient preference would be able to provide a definitive judgment about the balance. The NIH consensus guideline does not define its task this way. Instead, it says the task is "to identify the issues for which there are currently sufficient confirmed data," which appears to be quite independent of patient preferences/values or of weighing risks and benefits. Indeed, the document throughout reports screening and treatment interventions for which the research demonstrates no survival benefits.

Yet it seems to be weighing something when it produces recommendations: for example, it concludes that "this [level of risk] is probably not high enough to warrant prophylactic oophorectomy" (492), that "despite the absence of prospective data, this is sufficient risk for her to be screened" (492), and that "the risk of ovarian cancer . . . is sufficiently high" (493). In no case is "sufficient" defined.

Overall, the guideline's attitude toward patient preference is difficult to understand, in part because it accepts patient preferences that are inconsistent with the panel's conclusions about possible benefit. Initially, the guideline assures readers that the panel's conclusions are "based on the scientific evidence" (491). Thus, when the data show no benefits for screening women who have fewer than one risk factor for ovarian cancer, the guideline does not support such screening ("With current knowledge and technology, the benefits of screening a woman who has one or no first-degree relative with ovarian cancer are unproven" [492]). Yet, it says that screening should be offered if that is what the patient wants, as long as the woman has at least one "first-degree relative" as a risk factor. (This is justified, the guideline says, because "despite the absence of prospective data, this is sufficient risk for her to be screened" [492].)

Similarly, the panel reports that, after a woman has undergone a second relapse, several drugs have been used but "no survival benefit has been demonstrated by any of these regimens . . . patient preference for either vigorous treatment or no treatment should be respected" (495). These appear to be, contrary to the guideline's claim, standards that are not "based on the scientific evidence."

Clearly the panel is giving great weight to patient preferences in the absence of any scientific data showing benefit for the activities desired by the patients. It is possible that such conclusions arise from the panelists' sensing or considering benefits other than morbidity and mortality, such as providing the patient with psychological reassurance or earlier knowledge of disease that would enable life planning.[12] But if that is the case, the panel does not explain its thinking and tacitly seems to accept a consumer definition of medical appropriateness. That is, while claiming scientific authority, it is also claiming authority by endorsing patient choice.

A second part of this guideline's problematic approach to patients' values and preferences appears in the language and structure of some recommendations. For example, if the guideline exists to help caregivers clarify when and which treatment should be offered to women who may or do have ovarian cancer and to ensure that women have the information they need to decide about the offered treatment, then the guideline would reasonably talk in terms of what should be offered and even recommended. Sometimes this goal is clearly reflected in such phrases as "the recommended treatment for patients with low malignant potential ovarian tumors" (493). Such phrasing seems to say something like, "We, the members of this panel, believe that you physicians out there ought not just offer but should go so far as to recommend this treatment for patients with low malignant potential ovarian tumors." At other times, however, this sense of "offering" or of "recommending" treatment is supplanted by a more traditional language of physician authority: "All patients with grade 3 tumors *require* adjuvant therapy" (493; italics added). At other points, the patient disappears entirely, replaced only by the "adnexal mass" that "requires surgery." In these phrasings, the guideline's endorsement of patient involvement in decision making seems minimal.

Summary: NIH Guideline

Authority for this NIH Consensus Conference guideline is claimed on the grounds of both science and process, but these claims are not convincing. The text asserts but does not demonstrate high-quality evaluation and interpretation of the research data and asserts but does not demonstrate an open and unbiased process in the production of final recommendations. Furthermore, it claims both patient preference and scientific authority for decision making, even if the two are inconsistent.

American College of Physicians Guideline for Counseling Postmenopausal Women about Preventive Hormone Therapy[13]

Description of the ACP Guideline

This guideline is published under the name and the authority of the American College of Physicians through one of its committees and one of its subcommittees. The simultaneously published literature review, from which the guideline text is drawn, is published under the names of its eight authors. From these texts, it appears that the ACP's Subcommittee on Clinical Efficacy Assessment commissioned the preparation of the literature review under the supervision of a single physician (Grady). That physician enlisted seven others (three physicians, two PhDs, one MPH, and one MS) to prepare the literature review. The literature review including meta-analysis was then sent to eighteen outside reviewers from various medical specialties. The eight original authors then revised the literature review in response to these comments and submitted it to the ACP subcommittee that had commissioned it. The subcommittee, its parent Health and Public Policy Committee, and finally the ACP Board of Regents approved the literature review. It was then submitted for publication.

In a guideline footnote, we are told that the guideline was "authored" by Grady and three of the seven others who prepared the literature review as well as by one physician not involved in the literature review. Apparently, the guideline was not submitted either for review or for approval other than to the ACP Board of Regents. It includes numerical references to the literature review, identifying "support" for statements in the guideline.

Literature Review

The authors of the literature review provide detailed information on how they used the research literature to build a model that would enable them to quantify risks and benefits of hormone therapy. They use the active voice almost exclusively ("we reviewed," "we chose," "we calculated," "we estimated," "we repeated," etc.), making very clear that they are the ones who did this, not some nameless research assistants. They specify the task of the review: "to quantify the risks and benefits of hormone therapy in asymptomatic postmenopausal women."

Each section of the review begins with the achievement of the goal in one aspect of the question. Thus, for example, section 3.1, "Endometrial Cancer," begins, "A fifty-year-old woman has a 2.6 percent lifetime probability of developing cancer of the endometrium." Section 3.2, on breast cancer, begins, "[A] 50-year-old woman has a 10 percent lifetime probability of developing and a 3 percent probability of dying of breast cancer." The initial quantitative statement is then followed by a discussion of the research studies that lead the authors to their conclusion, and a summary statement that quantifies the risk factors (e.g., "In our model, we used the pooled relative risk of 0.96 for stroke among estrogen users and among estrogen plus progestin users"). The product of the review is very orderly and very precise in explaining how the authors proceeded, what conclusions they drew, and how they went about drawing those conclusions.

Connection between Data and Recommendations

The literature review connects statements in the review with the underlying literature although it does not in any way rate the quality of the underlying research, other than by the occasional use of such phrases as "some studies *suggest*" or "side-effects *appear* to be less problematic." The guideline appears to complete this connection both by drawing the specific guideline language directly from the literature review and by referencing the section of the literature review that provides further discussion of the guideline statement. The journal editors say that the reference numbers "support statements made here [in the guideline]," implying that the number will lead to the supporting research or outcomes literature. What it leads to, however, is the meta-analysis made by the authors. For example, the guideline recommendation that "[a]ll women, regardless of race, should consider preventive hormone therapy" sends the reader to section 6.6 of the literature review, which, in turn, provides a discussion of this recommendation but notes that most research studies on HRT have white women as subjects and thus there is no literature to cite, although tables relating to the meta-analysis are cited. Thus, there is a somewhat longer—and weaker—chain between the recommendations and the literature: guideline recommendation refers to author analysis/discussion refers to meta-analysis refers to research data to the extent that it exists.

Quantified Conclusions

The guideline and literature review authors provide extensive quantified conclusions, although of a different kind than those provided, for example, in the RAND guideline (to follow). Use of meta-analysis as well as a quantified goal means that the literature review provides tables that report conclusions such as this: a fifty-year-old white woman with a history of coronary artery disease and treated with long-term hormone replacement would be expected on average to have a 2.1 percent increase in life expectancy (from seventy-six years to seventy-seven years and seven months). This quantification would seem to lead naturally to fairly clear recommendations. Yet the authors conclude from this only that "hormone therapy *should probably* be recommended." It is not clear whether this hesitancy derives from the inadequacy of the research data (observational rather than randomized studies); from unwillingness to make a strong statement in light of the intended use of the guideline as a "counseling" tool for women, who should be allowed to make all decisions themselves; from fear that a stronger statement would undermine faith in the individual physician's clinical judgment; or from fear that it might establish an undesired standard of care. Whatever the reason, the guideline authors and sponsors appear to back away from the quantified conclusions that they have expended considerable effort to achieve.

Formal Method

The guideline recommendations are said to flow directly from the meta-analysis, and thus there seems to be no need for a process at the level of interpretation. If that were the case, it is somewhat difficult to explain why the literature review had eight authors and the guidelines five authors (nine individual authors in total).

Nevertheless, what appears in the literature review, it is said, is what appears in the guidelines. Yet the guideline includes five recommendations while the literature review includes only three conclusions. The difference lies in the guideline recommendation that "all women, regardless of race, should consider preventive hormone therapy" (not stated as such in the literature review) and the recommendation that "the risks of hormone therapy may outweigh its benefits in women who are at increased risk for breast cancer." In the literature review, the latter statement is not made. Rather, the text says simply that for that group "the decision regarding hormone therapy is difficult," and then proceeds to explain that difficulty.

Inclusiveness and Selection Procedures

Unlike the AHCPR and RAND guidelines, which go to great lengths to identify the panel that created the guidelines and to justify their selection, the ACP guideline seems to derive its authority not from its authors but from the ACP itself. Indeed, the "authors" of the guideline are named only in a footnote. (The ACP's name is on the author line, but in the footnote the five are said to have "authored" the guideline.) Further, although the members of the ACP committee and subcommittee are listed in the same footnote, they are identified only by name and degree, and not by institution or specialty.

The subcommittee is said to have "commissioned" the writing of the literature review and guideline to Dr. Grady, but the text does not explain how that commissioning worked nor how Dr. Grady then chose her seven colleagues (from three different institutions in San Francisco). We are not told anything about the subspecialty orientation of the physicians involved in "authoring" the materials nor of the members of the committee and subcommittee that commissioned and reviewed the material. Thus, this guideline does not use information about authors/panelists in order to claim expertise and inclusiveness. Nor are claims made about patient or public involvement in the process. Despite the fact that hormone replacement therapy is an important issue for women, the authors were limited to academic health care and health policy professionals, four of whom are women. The inference that might be drawn is that the heart of the process was the meta-analysis, which required expertise. The guideline presents only an institutional face.

Public Nature of the Process

The guideline is not presented as a publicly informed document. Indeed, even to the extent that it was made available to others for comment, the "others" are unidentified and are only said to be from medical specialties other than internal medicine.

Breadth of Dissemination

Dissemination is through journal publication. Although the guideline itself is short and could be edited and recast as a patient information document, there was apparently no intention to do so. This may be all the more surprising considering that the guideline recommendations emphasize so strongly that all postmenopausal women should consider hormone replacement therapy and that the decision will require considerable patient education because the guideline recommendations are so minimal. (The guideline can best be summarized thus: women without uteri and women with or at increased risk of coronary artery disease "are likely to benefit from estrogen therapy" although "[f]or other women, the best course of action is not clear.")

Patient Preferences

The guideline recommendations are so tentative that unlimited patient preference should be the result of any treatment decision, but there are no built-in patient preference considerations in the guideline.

Summary: ACP Guidelines

This guideline is puzzling in many respects. The authority of the guideline appears to lie in its science, in the meta-analysis's connection to the research literature and to the guideline conclusions. The guideline conclusions, however, are so weak as to undo the importance of the connection. In addition, the guideline (which is only four pages long, half of which are occupied by tables and exhibits) begins by stating that the research literature is inadequate to make the kind of quantifiable conclusions that the guidelines are based upon. Although that is typical of research quality at this time, acknowledging it so directly tends to undercut the authority of the guidelines. It is for this reason, presumably, that many guidelines emphasize their process, and particularly their inclusiveness. This ACP guideline undercuts its potential authority at virtually every opportunity, making it problematic with respect to authority for physicians, patients, courts, and insurers.

The desire to convey more than is strictly justified by the science, however, appears at certain points. For example, the central problem of hormone replacement therapy is that it requires dealing with three factors simultaneously: the risk of endometrial and breast cancer from the treatment, the prevention of coronary disease and hip fracture by the treatment, and treatment burdens. Because the research is inadequate, it is difficult to be sure about the probability of risks and benefits, though the treatment burdens are well identified. Thus, a decision inevitably entails balancing all three factors. Patients will be the best authority on how that balance will be weighed in their own lives. The guideline generally defers to this patient balancing, especially when the research is very weak. But the guideline makes an exception in recommendation 4, which says, "The risks of hormone therapy may outweigh its benefits in women who are at increased risk for breast cancer." If this statement is true, then it is also true that "the risks of hormone therapy may *not* outweigh its benefits in women who are at increased risk for breast cancer." If so, the guideline recommendation might more properly read, "The risks of hormone therapy may or may not outweigh its benefits in women who are at increased risk for breast cancer." Another way of saying that is, "We don't know if women who are at increased risk for breast cancer should have hormone therapy." Because the final recommendation is just that ("For other women, the best course of action is unclear"), the decision to slant the recommendation toward not using the treatment is puzzling.

RAND Corporation: Cataract Surgery: A Literature Review and Ratings of Appropriateness and Cruciality[14]

Description of RAND Guideline

RAND guidelines use a nine-physician panel in a formal and easily replicable method (the method, not necessarily the results, are replicable). In order to quantify panelists' judgments about the appropriateness of specific treatment in a great variety of clinical circumstances, each panelist rates the treatment in question on a scale of 1–9 for potentially hundreds of different clinical presentations. The responses are quantified and translated into "indicators" of "appropriate," "inappropriate," and "uncertain" treatment use in each circumstance. The physicians on the panel are "guided" by a literature review produced by RAND researchers. The panelists also engage in a formal process ("Delphi process") in which they discuss the panel's aggregate ratings. This is used to encourage some move toward consensus after the first round. Two or more rounds of ratings are then scored. The final product takes these considered ratings and turns them into numerical scores indicating whether treatment is appropriate, inappropriate, or uncertain in each clinical circumstance.

Literature Review

It is generally said that the weakest link in the RAND method is the uncertain link between outcomes data and the panelists' judgments.[15] By contrast, the NIH also prepares a background literature review (bibliography and selected abstracts) for its conferees. But the conferees are actually present when the witnesses present their interpretations of the literature and are able to discuss conclusions and inferences with them. The RAND process does not provide such an opportunity. Thus, although an extensive literature review is prepared by RAND researchers, reviewed by members of specialty societies, and then sent to the panelists in advance of their first ratings round (in the case of cataract surgery, they rated indications three separate times for appropriateness/inappropriateness and twice for "cruciality"), there is no way to guarantee that the panelists actually read the literature review or that they are influenced by the conclusions it provides.

The RAND literature review (unlike the NIH literature review) is published, in company with the appropriateness indications. The cataract surgery literature review is extensive (296 articles from 1980 to 1990 were selected from almost 2,380 "full-text articles" that were reviewed for inclusion) and is divided into separate issues (e.g., efficacy, risks and complications). The quality of the studies reported is assessed. For example, when reporting upon efficacy, the authors note that only one study was prospective and randomized and that most are "uncontrolled, observational studies." In the conclusion to this section, they note that the common outcomes measure of available studies is visual acuity but that patients' functional vision would be a better outcomes measure. "Thus, in view of the predominantly observational study designs, summary descriptive statistics should be interpreted with caution" (p. 25). Such a conclusion, of course, may lead panelists to believe that they can safely ignore the literature review because it will not give them any clear guidance.

Connection between Data and Recommendations

By coupling publication of its literature review and its panelists' conclusions, the RAND guideline suggests a link between the two that is ultimately unjustified. The literature review is produced by one group and the appropriateness indicators by another. The link is not made by including in the publication a postpanel assessment of how the appropriateness conclusions and the research conclusions match. This link has, however, been made in other RAND guideline projects. In studying appropriateness indicators for carotid endarterectomy, the authors conclude that "the physicians' indications and ratings were consistent with those in the literature, and statistical analysis demonstrated that they followed logical clinical rationale."[16] Readers of the cataract guideline do not have this assurance. Unless they also carefully read the literature review, they will be unable to find whether or when there are instances (like those in the NIH guideline on ovarian cancer screening) in which procedures are judged appropriate in the absence of data that would justify the conclusion.

Quantified Conclusions

Although the RAND process relies very heavily on quantified conclusions, it is not the research literature that provides them. Instead, it is the process that provides quantified conclusions. Indeed, this quantified process may be the most important part of the RAND guidelines with respect to their claim to be authoritative because it creates the only replicable process and produces quantifiable conclusions. (See IV.C.1, "Process Method.")

Process Method

The cataract guideline describes the process in considerable detail, including its limitations and potential for ambiguity. For example, noting that the use of a nine-point scale implies equal intervals, the authors discuss the problems of anchoring in their scale (although the center "is well-anchored at the point where risk equals benefit" and the end points are "anchored to some degree," a four-point difference is bigger than a one-point but not necessarily four times as large) (p. 47). A table is provided to offer insight into the degree of agreement among panelists for any particular indication for cataract surgery (the panel rated, on a scale of 1–9, almost 3,000 different indications). Because the final conclusions of appropriateness, inappropriateness, and uncertainty rest on the degree of panel agreement, the authors are careful to explain how and why they defined "agreement" (they used a statistical definition in order to permit replicability with different numbers of panel members). In the eight pages used to describe the panel methodology in the text, the authors provide four separate tables (using approximately two and one-half pages) to clarify the methodology.

No other guideline reviewed here devoted as much attention to explaining how it did what it did. This is important because, although all four of these guidelines are ultimately completed in private and in that private process lies considerable potential for unfairness, the entire RAND process is done in private. Indeed, the panelists' judgments of appropriateness are made alone and independently. No panelist knows for certain how any other panelist "voted." Even after publication of the results, panelists can know how others rated the procedure only if there was unanimity. This careful description of the process lends authority to the product because it is so specific, because it tries to minimize domination of some panelists by others, and because it is replicable.

The description may imply that the process is reliable in terms of replicability. And although it is true that the method is replicable and, in that sense, is reliable, nothing can be said thereby as to the reliability of the conclusions. That is, if the method were applied in exactly the same manner using nine different panelists, the results might (or might not) be different. Indeed, RAND researchers have shown that specialist and generalist physicians as well as physicians from different countries judge indications differently for the same procedure.[17] Given the practice variation rates in the use of some procedures in the United States, it is certainly possible that similar differences would be found for different panelists even if they were from the same background and geographical representation as the current panelists.

Inclusiveness and Selection Procedures

The cataract guideline's authors are careful to describe not only who sat upon the panel ("nationally recognized experts") but how they were chosen and how representative they are. The procedure they report is to ask specialty societies (American Academy of Family Physicians, American Academy of Ophthalmology, American College of Physicians, American Geriatrics Society, and American Society of Cataract and Refractive Surgery) to nominate from their own groups proposed panel members. Upon receipt of these nominations, panelists "*were chosen*" and "*were selected*." In a document notable for use of the active voice (in contrast to much scientific writing), the cataract guideline leaves a blank as to who did the choosing and the selecting, suggesting that the panelists were chosen by some inevitable process or arrived full-blown from the ear of Zeus. The use of the passive voice at this point suggests that no one wanted to take full responsibility for the final selection process.

Whoever did this selecting from an unknown—because unspecified—number of nominees based his/her judgment on "clinical expertise, community influence (e.g. in professional organizations), and geographic location." The selection, it is said, "represented academic and community practice and different specialties," but it does not say that this was, in fact, the basis of selection. Of the three specific selection factors (clinical expertise, community influence, and geographic location), only the last can be judged from the document itself. One might think that geographic location would, as a selection factor, be used to select members from different geographical areas. The nine panelists, however, include two from Texas, two from Maryland, three from the West Coast, and three (including the two from Maryland) from the East Coast. No panelist is from the Midwest. The claim is made that "all four major census regions were represented" in this selection, which sounds impressive but perhaps means only that if you divide the United States in quarters, each quarter will contain at least one of these physicians. All four major census regions would also be represented if the panel included one physician each from Boston, Tennessee, and Texas and six physicians from UCLA. The larger question, of course, would be whether geographical representation makes a difference, especially in the face of the guideline's literature review report that current practice variation levels are not high. The geographic-balance claim can only be understood as a way of making a fairness claim for authority. The specialty selection appears to reflect the claimed balance; the panel members include five ophthalmologists (four who perform cataracts and one who does not), two internists, a geriatrician, and a family practice physician. (For guidelines on an ophthalmologic procedure, a majority of the panelists would legitimately be expected to be ophthalmologists.)

Public Nature of Process
The RAND guidelines are conducted outside public view.

Breadth of Dissemination
The RAND guidelines are notable for their apparent disinterest in dissemination, let alone broad dissemination. The explanatory material in the formal summary of the guideline does not mention either for whom the guideline is intended or why cataract surgery was chosen as a subject. Published as a 300-page book by RAND, this guideline is not distributed by academic or commercial publishers. It cannot realistically be published in a medical journal (as the NIH Consensus Conference statements and the ACP guidelines are and as the AHCPR guidelines could be) because of its scope and size. For example, judgments of appropriateness for cataract surgery are made for several thousand different clinical presentations. Thus, judgments of appropriateness differ for the patient (1) with unilateral cataract and other ocular disease; (2) who has branch retinal vein occlusion without macular involvement; (3) whose best corrected visual acuity in contralateral eye is 20/50–20/70; (4) who expresses difficulty with recreation, watching TV, or reading; and (5) whose best corrected visual acuity before surgery in the operated eye is 20/50–20/70, as compared to the patient who has the same first four characteristics listed but whose best corrected visual acuity before surgery in the operate eye is 20/80–20/100 (p. 212). Over 200 pages of the text of this publication are devoted to appropriateness ratings for the many possible combinations of clinical presentations. The guideline is simply silent as to its audience.

Role of Patient Preferences

Patient preferences are not incorporated in the clinical indicators, although it could be argued that the final "uncertain" category is one in which clinicians should be particularly scrupulous about engaging patients to explore their values, because these are areas in which the relationship between burdens and benefits is unclear to the physicians. Although many of the listed indicators speak to patients' assessments of their condition (e.g., the patient has difficulty driving or watching TV, or with ADLs or employment, or complains of glare), these are not in and of themselves indications of appropriateness of surgery. For example, if a patient with a specified clinical presentation reports difficulty driving, the appropriateness of cataract surgery would depend not on the patient's complaint but upon the "best corrected visual acuity before surgery in the operated eye" (81). That is, the appropriateness of the surgery depends upon a measurement category, not upon the patient's belief that a surgical correction is preferable to an eyeglass correction when it comes to having difficulty driving.

Even though patient preferences play no role, quality-of-life judgments appear to be important, insofar as there are two major categories (patients with life expectancy of less than six months and patients with severe dementia) in which appropriateness judgments vary considerably. That is, patients who are not severely demented and who are not terminally ill but who have the same visual problems and functional problems as patients who are severely demented or who are terminally ill frequently have higher appropriateness ratings under numerous circumstances. For example, there are four different sets of clinical circumstances in which the median appropriateness rating for cataract surgery for terminally ill patients is 7, for severely demented patients 2–5, and for nondemented, nonterminally ill patients 8–9. (pp. 53–57) (9= very appropriate, 1=very inappropriate). This means that for the demented patients, cataract surgery would be inappropriate; for the terminally ill and nondemented, nonterminally ill patients, cataract surgery would be considered appropriate. The only difference among these patients is their life expectancy or their mental status. Thus, the differences in scoring reflect judgments about the value of cataract surgery for demented patients simply because of their dementia. This might be understood as a lack of concern for patient values.

Summary: RAND Guidelines

This absence of attention to both broad dissemination and to patient preferences and the unexplained use of quality-of-life judgments suggest that the authority of these guidelines lies in their professional source, their professional application, and their reliable and quantified process. They are created by physicians for physicians and based upon physicians' values. This is a vastly different authority claim from that suggested, e.g., by AHCPR with its emphasis on dissemination to the lay public and its inclusion of members of the public on its panels, or by NIH and ACP with their deference to patient preferences in the absence of justifying data. The RAND guidelines present themselves as exclusive rather than inclusive, as proprietary rather than public, as "scientific" (based on their *process* methodology) rather than as process- or consensus-driven with all the political implications of those phrases. Their "science" may be questionable, of course, as in the implication that panelist representation from four major census areas would lead to superior results, or that the panelists' judgments reflect the literature review, or that the panel process's numerical results are both valid and reliable, but it is the authority of science, quantitativeness, and medial expertise that informs the product.

Agency for Health Care Policy and Research (AHCPR): Otitis Media with Effusion Guideline[18]

Description of AHCPR Guideline

This seventy-four-page guideline was published in 1994 by a U.S. government agency whose task is to produce practice guidelines. The descriptive material is largely cast in the passive voice, and it is difficult to understand exactly how the guideline was created. Apparently, AHCPR gave a contract to the American Academy of Pediatrics to create the guideline. The Academy worked in concert with a consortium (the American Academy of Family Physicians and the American Academy of Otolaryngology—Head and Neck Surgery). The consortium "convened a panel" of nineteen members with AHCPR's approval. The American Academy or the consortium subcontracted the literature review to the Children's Hospital of Pittsburgh. Prior to the literature review's completion, the consortium held an open meeting to seek out the views of other health care professionals. After the data were analyzed, draft guidelines were prepared, sent out for both peer and "pilot reviews," and revised in the light of these reviews.

The guideline is addressed to practitioners ("The purpose . . . is to assist those who provide health care to young children" [p. 3]), although in a preface to the guideline, the AHCPR administrator says the guidelines are intended "to assist practitioner *and* patient decisions" (italics added). The guideline has a fairly narrow focus (what to do with otitis media with effusion [OME] in children between the ages of one and three who have no other significant problems). It offers some specific answers about recommended therapies over three time frames and then suggests that individual clinical judgment and parental guidance direct the actual decision.

The preface introduces the guideline as both scientifically authoritative and only potentially helpful. On the one hand, the conclusions derive from "explicit, science-based methods and expert clinical judgment," are "primarily based on the published scientific literature," and "reflect the state of knowledge, current at the time of publication, on effective and appropriate care." On the other hand, "recommendations may not be appropriate for use in all circumstances. Decisions to adopt any particular recommendation must be made by the practitioner in light of available resources and circumstances presented by individual patients." This deference to clinicians and patient/parents is echoed in the "Executive Summary," wherein the "Panel recognizes the clinical circumstances of individual patients can require additional judgment of health care providers and parents regarding therapy." That is, the guideline contains only general statements to be modified by each practitioner and parent as they judge best, despite the scientific expertise that created them.

Literature Review

According to the OME guideline, the panel "based their approach to guideline development on AHCPR recommendations and the principles of Eddy."[19] The "principles of [David] Eddy" may simply be a part of AHCPR recommendations insofar as we are told that the "Panel was introduced to Eddy's principles . . . at its first two meetings."[20] We are not told who performed the introduction. Without further specifying what belonged to Eddy and what belonged to AHCPR, the methodology, as described, involved first specifying the clinical question and then "developing literature search strategies, examining the literature critically, and developing evidence tables based on the data extracted from the literature review."

The literature review focused on categorizing the quality of evidence demonstrated in published research studies. Then each panel subcommittee decided what quality of research would be accepted for review on its topic. For example, "the subcommittees examining pharmaceutical or surgical interventions accepted only randomized, blinded, controlled studies for inclusion." (This standard—a high one for surgical interventions—should be contrasted with the RAND cataract surgery guideline description of its evidence: "There were no randomized, controlled, double blind trials" [p. v]). Although the panelists determined the standard of adequacy, the literature search itself was subcontracted (to Children's Hospital of Pittsburgh).

The bibliographic search, we are told, was extensive, using multiple databases and search strategies. The literature review method required judging whether an article met the standard specified by the panel. If the article did, then two people independently abstracted data in order to ensure accuracy. Because there had been a contentious issue at Children's Hospital of Pittsburgh involving faculty doing research on otitis media with effusion and the effectiveness of antibiotic treatment, all research studies authored by those with a connection to the University of Pittsburgh as well as research studies involving antibiotic treatment of OME were reviewed by independent reviewers. When possible, meta-analysis was conducted.

The description of this literature review exudes confidence about both the complexity of the task and the diligence with which it was pursued to ensure that conclusions could be safely based on the research evidence. Indeed, at one point, the panel is reported to have "conducted an additional literature search and evaluation,"[21] suggesting that these busy professionals were not only attending periodic meetings in Washington but also contacting colleagues for literature references and subsequently abstracting articles.

Connection between Data and Recommendations

According to the text, the "*Guideline* is based on the relevant scientific literature and on the Panel's expert clinical opinion."[22] Additionally, "other sources of input into the Guideline included the Panel's own expertise, information from Open Meeting presentations, peer and pilot reviewer comments, and Panel subcommittee analysis of the literature."[23] These descriptions suggest a process that is not consistent with the description of the literature review. That is, the literature review is described as being so rigorous that one is inclined to believe that it will, on its own, answer the vital questions. The panel was generally able, it says, to distinguish through this process among high-quality scientific evidence, good-quality scientific evidence, limited scientific evidence, no scientific evidence, and compelling evidence (p. 8). But the panel admits to the break in the link between science and recommendations: "Of note is that the final recommendations are at least partially subjective; . . . judgments about the quality of the science could not be fully objective." Panelists disagreed about how to interpret the evidence and, in the absence of evidence, were inclined to depend on theoretical arguments.

Quantified Conclusions

The panel developed levels of recommendation (strong, moderate, and plain) based on the quality of the evidence, the consensus of the panel, or the expert opinion of the panel. The document does not describe how the last two standards differ. In addition, the panel uses two other categories: clinical options and no recommendation. Clinical options involve situations where there is no "compelling scientific evidence" (the document does not explain how "compelling scientific evidence" differs from either "high-quality" or "good-quality" or even "limited" scientific evidence). "No recommendations" are made "when scientific evidence is lacking" and there is "no compelling reason" to make a recommendation. What constitutes a "compelling" reason is as unexplained as what constitutes "compelling scientific evidence."

Thus, although the panel creates through this complex method levels of recommendations based upon levels of scientific evidence, it fails to define a number of the key terms. Furthermore, in addressing twenty-one distinct questions in regard to OME, it ultimately makes only eight recommendations. Of these eight, five recommend against intervention (e.g., tonsillectomy, steroids, decongestants, adenoidectomy) and three recommend intervention (e.g., hearing evaluation). Four of the eight are "strong recommendations" (two are based on "evidence," but despite the panel's efforts to grade evidence, no grade is specified for the evidence upon which these two recommendations are made; one is a "strong recommendation based on evidence that can be generalized," another undefined term; and two are based on limited evidence). There is one moderate recommendation based on limited evidence, and there are three plain recommendations based on limited evidence (again, despite the categorizations of high-quality, good-quality, and absent evidence, the panel uses the phrase "limited evidence," a phrase they have not previously defined: is it limited high-quality evidence or limited good-quality evidence?). After these eight recommendations, there are thirteen "options" or "no recommendations," which leave clinicians to do whatever they or the parents choose, just as they did before there were any guidelines.

The bottom line in this attempt to quantify through sharp definitions the quality of evidence on which the guideline recommendations are based is that with two exceptions, nothing is based on the scientific evidence and everything is based upon the expert opinion. This is not meant to criticize the panel, of course, because where there is no scientific data, no data can provide grounding for recommendations. But the AHCPR guideline places great emphasis on its methods for evaluating outcomes data, for incorporating them into the recommendations, and for justifying its recommendations. Unfortunately, the product does not sustain the claim.

Formal Method

Once the literature review was completed, the panel held multiple meetings. We are told who chaired the meetings (the cochairs and the "methodologist"), that consensus on each question was sought, and that panelists voted if consensus failed. A successful vote on a recommendation required that at least fifteen of nineteen support it (or may have required that no more than four people be opposed to it; quorum rules are not described). The guideline also acknowledges the presence of minority views, which sometimes led to minority reports that are included in an appendix to the guideline "Technical Report."[24]

Inclusiveness and Selection Procedures

The AHCPR guideline panel was drawn primarily from nominations provided by specialty organizations. After the consortium selected a group of fifteen, those names were published in the *Federal Register* and sent to the nominating organizations for response. This resulted in eighteen more nominations, four of whom were added to the panel, giving it a final total of nineteen. Balance was sought in terms of expertise, geography, race, and gender. The nineteen panel members included one consumer representative, three nurses, eleven physicians, and four PhDs—ten women and nine men. The consumer representative (a woman) is a freelance writer from Washington, D.C. The geographical balance does better by the Midwest than the RAND panel did (two members of the panel are from Michigan). Although there is no a priori reason to suppose that race, gender, or geography would affect recommendations, attention to such detail (and careful recounting of it) suggests a belief that such issues will help to provide authority for the guideline. Surprisingly, in a guideline on OME, no panelist was qualified by virtue of being a parent.

Public Nature of Process

Like the NIH statement, the AHCPR guideline refers several times to the conducting of an open session, apparently emphasizing that this was not a closed-shop operation. Prior to the completion of the literature review, for example, the panel held "an Open Meeting that was announced in the *Federal Register*."[25] In the foreword to the document, the panel notes that it did not depend solely on the data but also upon "information from Open Meeting presentations [presumably the one held in connection with the literature review, despite the use of the plural 'presentations'], peer and pilot reviewer comments." At no point, however, is this open meeting explained (neither where it was held, nor who was invited, nor who attended), nor is there any attempt to show how the open meeting specifically affected the results.

Breadth of Dissemination

AHCPR guidelines are the most widely disseminated of any of the four. They are printed in different forms by AHCPR: they are written for clinicians (a quick guide and the full guideline) and for parents/patients; they are available on the Internet; and they are available without charge by writing to AHCPR. Patient versions of the guidelines are directed at patient education but, arguably, also intended to accustom the public to the very idea of guidelines. The breadth of dissemination increases the guidelines' authority, however, because patient/parents who arrive in their pediatricians' offices have an additional source of authority with which to challenge the doctor.

Patient Preferences

Although AHCPR included a patient representative in its guideline, parents do not have a strong presence, with one exception: the issue of environmental-risk control. On this issue, based on limited scientific evidence but panel consensus, the physician is advised to counsel parents about three environmental-risk factors that the parents control. Parents may not be pleased, however, with the role given to them. The first, propped-bottle feeding for infants, lacks relevance because the guideline is directed at one- to three-year-olds, who would not have propped bottles. The second, passive smoke, is an add-on. Because passive cigarette smoke is known to be detrimental to other child health issues, the risk of OME "should be added to the many other reasons" that parents should stop smoking, even in the absence of evidence about its relationship to OME. The third environmental-risk factor about which parents should be counseled is their child's participation in "group child care" (i.e, day care). Grouping it with the other two implies that it is an easily modified lifestyle factor, hardly the case for working parents who have children in day care. Thus, the guidelines seem to take this as an opportunity to lean on parents in order to get them to stop doing things that pediatricians disapprove of, regardless of the activities' relationship to OME in one- to three-year-olds or the parents' ability to change them.

On the other hand, the guideline gives considerable scope to choice about pursuing various interventions (e.g., observation or antibiotic therapy), and the guideline could at least be interpreted as offering parents (rather than physicians) the opportunity to make that choice. That is a particularly legitimate interpretation in the face of AHCPR's dissemination materials, which provide in essence the same information to parents and physicians about these choices.

Summary: AHCPR Guideline

One of the most striking aspects of the AHCPR guideline is its interest in distancing itself from the government. The OME guideline is referred to in the preface as one of the "AHCPR-assisted clinical guidelines" and elsewhere, with some small variation, as the "Otitis Media with Effusion Guideline." By contrast, the Consensus Conference guideline is routinely referred to as an "NIH Consensus Conference Statement."

Except in the preface (where it is done only in a generic sense), AHCPR's name is not connected to the guideline. In the document itself, it appears as the publisher, under the auspices of the Department of Health and Human Services (DHHS). DHHS, however, in bold print warns readers that just because it published these guidelines, it doesn't necessarily believe in them ("Publication of this guideline does not necessarily represent endorsement by the U.S. Department of Health and Human Services"). Within the text, at some points the guideline seems to be the property of the American Academy of Pediatrics, which coordinated the work under contract from AHCPR. At others, it seems to be the property of "the Consortium" (which is apparently composed of two specialty groups, the American Academy of Family Physicians and the American Academy of Otolaryngology—Head and Neck Surgery, but may also include the American Academy of Pediatrics). It is somewhat difficult to determine from the "Executive Summary" who did what because, although the contract was with the American Academy of Pediatrics, it was the consortium that convened the panel. This work, however, was scarcely independent of AHCPR: the agency chose the topic and chose the methods that were to be used in developing the guideline (the actual phrase is "recommended," but one is doubtful about whether the Academy would have been awarded the "contract" had it been interested in using some other method), and finally, the convening of the panel was done "with AHCPR approval." It is again unclear whether AHCPR approved the convening or the appointment of the panel members, but in either case, AHCPR was central to the task of producing a guideline. In the "Executive Summary," the panel is said to have "applied the AHCPR's recommended methods," suggesting a rather mechanical process—which, in the world of guidelines methodology, can scarcely be an accurate description.

One can, of course, only speculate on this language and what it means about the guidelines and about AHCPR's role. At the very least it seems to suggest that AHCPR wants to take credit, as a result of its deep involvement in the guidelines process, for ensuring fairness by supervising vested interests and, at the same time, to take credit for its noninvolvement in the guidelines, thereby promising that the government's heavy hand did not influence the process. The various phrasings in the guidelines used to explain both the audience for, and the basis and use of, the OME guidelines suggest that there are multiple and potentially inconsistent goals that are to be achieved by the guidelines. They are authoritative because they are scientific, but they are not so authoritative that they would override clinical or parental judgment; they are intended to improve the quality of care, and they are intended to reduce costs; they are the product of the private sector, but they are centrally shaped by the government; they are for physicians, and they are for parents; they are to guide, and they are to assist. The OME guidelines, strong on method and weak on authoritative conclusions, have something for everyone.

Conclusion

These guidelines wrestle with the problem of authority in different ways. In two, the attempt to provide authoritative guidelines seems to be a central concern; in the other two, it is an issue, but there appears to be more conflict around it. The RAND and the NIH guidelines seem to be trying to present an authoritative face although in very different ways. In the case of the AHCPR and the ACP guidelines, there seems more of an internal conflict about whether the goal is a guideline that provides authoritative direction for physicians and patients or, in the case of the ACP guideline, a guideline that maximizes the opportunity for patients to be in control of treatment decisions (offer treatment to everyone and let them decide because no decision is ever obviously correct) and, in the case of the AHCPR guideline, a guideline that maximizes the opportunity for individual physicians to guide treatment decisions (don't do some things but otherwise do—or offer—what seems appropriate to you as an individual physician).

Third-party payers will find the RAND and the NIH guidelines much easier to use as a basis for reimbursement, however, just because they offer a more authoritative presentation. It would be consummately easy for third-party payers to decide to use the appropriateness indicators as a basis for determining when to certify or to reimburse for cataract surgery. Although the NIH guideline would not translate quite as easily, the links between research and treatment decisions that are made, if not always honored, could also be codified fairly easily. By contrast, nothing could be drawn from the ACP and very little from the AHCPR guidelines to guide either utilization or reimbursement decisions.

None of the four guidelines is without an appeal to authority that the text shows is ultimately lacking; claims for process authority of inclusiveness are particularly notable in that respect, but the claims for substantive authority based on the connection between research and recommendations are also weak. Some might argue that guidelines should not be presented as very authoritative just because there is not sufficient evidence in most instances to provide authoritative guidelines. But that is to reenter the argument between Peto and Brook alluded to at the beginning of this paper: Should expert opinion be allowed to count as data? And if so, what constitutes an expert, and who chooses them?

RAND accepts the inevitable weakness of the data, apparently, and thus does not make a very strong attempt to connect it to the recommendations/conclusions. Instead it depends upon a strong process method to create both definite recommendations and a restraining force on the potential problems of ill-defined expertise. ACP, on the other hand, accepts the inadequacy of expertise. It pushes the data as far as it can, but then concludes that it cannot say much by way of recommendations. The NIH guideline, by contrast, seems unaware of the problems either of undefined expertise or of inadequate data. It is as if the panel were operating on the confidence levels of an earlier time in which professionals simply did the best they could, operating on a legitimate assumption of trust and good will. Finally, AHCPR, the newest player on the guideline block, takes an opposite tack to NIH: it seems aware of, but unfazed by, weak data and undefined expertise. Yet combining its acceptance of both, it ultimately seems able to make very little of either.

Guideline development is in its earliest stage, so it is hard to predict where it will go next. Eddy noted in 1993 that one of the three central questions of health care reform involved "how much evidence is needed to say that a treatment is 'appropriate,' that it should be used, and that it should be paid for."[26] Guideline development is still working on that first question. In a culture that highly values individualism and individual judgment, it may be near impossible to insist upon a more communitarian approach that says, in effect, "Even though we do not have perfect (or even near-perfect) research data that tell us what works, when it works, and why it works, we must make some general decisions that everyone—patients and physicians and insurers—will agree to follow." Until guideline development is seen within such a communitarian framework, the question of authority will remain unresolved, and unjustified authority claims will doubtless continue to be made.

A decision about what evidence should be considered authoritative can be made by professionals or by the public. If we no longer trust professionals to make it or if they are unwilling or unable to speak in a single voice, we will need to make it in the public forum. The public appears ill prepared, largely unaware of practice variations and of the unscientific nature of most treatment decision making. Education must then precede public discussion. A worrisome question, however, is whether Americans are open to such education. Do they want to learn about substantial practice variations? About harms resulting from overtreatment? About the use of unproven treatments that cause harms? About the great degree of medical uncertainty that is at play in all medical decisions? Or are they more interested in focusing solely on potential benefits? Would they prefer simply to accept the claim that the United States has the best health care system in the world, with the implicit and sometimes explicit promise that medical miracles are waiting for them behind every hospital door?

To understand why we must make a considered judgment about what constitutes authority requires us first to understand something about the dark side of medicine and the complexity of policy decisions. Then we will need to accept that many positions about authority have merit, even if we cannot adopt them all simultaneously. Until then, however, authority will continue to be asserted with rhetoric more than with conviction.

NOTES

1. M. R. Chassin et al., "Does Inappropriate Use Explain Geographic Variations in the Use of Health Care Services?" *JAMA* 258 (1987): 2533–7.

2. C. E. Phelps, correspondence, "Appropriateness Studies," *NEJM* 330, no. 6 (1994): 433–4.

3. R. H. Fletcher and S. W. Fletcher, editorial, "Clinical Practice Guidelines," *Annals of Internal Medicine* 113, no. 9 (1990): 645–6.

4. D. M. Eddy, "Practice Policies—What Are They?" *JAMA* 263, no. 6 (1990): 877–80.

5. R. H. Brook, "Practice Guidelines and Practicing Medicine: Are They Compatible?" *JAMA* 262, no. 21 (1989): 3027–30.

6. P. Cotton, "Medical News and Perspectives: Determining More Good Than Harm Is Not Easy," *JAMA* 270, no. 2 (1993): 153–8.

7. P. Cotton, "Medical News and Perspectives."

8. NIH Consensus Development Panel on Ovarian Cancer, "Ovarian Cancer: Screening, Treatment, and Follow-Up," *JAMA* 273, no. 6 (1995): 491–7.

9. The remaining two physicians are apparently in private practice in Maryland, and the previously mentioned attorney is with a private foundation in Maryland.

10. N. Roche and P. Durieux, "Clinical Practice Guidelines: From Methodological to Practical Issues," *Intensive Care Medicine* 20 (1994): 593–601.

11. N. Roche and P. Durieux, "Clinical Practice Guidelines," p. 594.

12. G. Povar, "Profiling and Performance Measures. What are the Ethical Issues?" *Medical Care* 33 (1 Suppl.) (1995): J560–8.

13. Published in *Annals of Internal Medicine* 117 (1992): 1038–41; "Hormone Replacement Therapy to Prevent Disease and Prolong Life in Postmenopausal Women," *Annals of Internal Medicine* 117, no. 2 (1992): 1016–37.

14. By P. P. Lee et al. (Santa Monica, Calif.: RAND, 1993), JRA-06.

15. N. Roche and P. Durieux, "Clinical Practice Guidelines."

70   Part II: Outcomes Data

16. N. J. Merrick et al., "Derivation of Clinical Indications for Carotid Endarterectomy by an Expert Panel," *Am J Publ Health* 77, no. 2 (1992): 187–90.

17. L. L. Leape et al., "Group Judgments of Appropriateness: The Effect of Panel Composition," *Quality Assurance Health Care* 4, no. 2 (1992): 151–9; R. H. Brook et al., "The Diagnosis and Treatment of Coronary Disease in Two Cultures: A Comparison of Doctors' Attitudes in the USA and the UK," *Lancet* (April 2, 1988): 1–11.

18. *Clinical Practice Guidelines,* Number 12 (Rockville, MD: USDHHS, 1994).

19. D. M. Eddy, "Practice Policies."

20. D. M. Eddy, "Practice Policies."

21. P. Cotton, "Medical News and Perspectives."

22. M. R. Chassin, "Does Inappropriate Use Explain Geographic Variations?"

23. M. R. Chassin, "Does Inappropriate Use Explain Geographic Variations?"; C. E. Phelps, "Appropriateness Studies."

24. *Clinical Practice Guidelines,* Number 12 (Rockville, MD: USDHHS, 1994).

25. P. Cotton, "Medical News and Perspectives."

26. D. M. Eddy, "Three Battles to Watch in the 1990s," *JAMA* 270, no. 4 (1993): 520–6.

Larry Culpepper and Jane Sisk

The Development of Practice Guidelines: A Case Study of Otitis Media with Effusion

Introduction

The development of clinical-practice guidelines has received high priority from public and private policy makers seeking to improve the quality of care and to contain costs. Federal guideline activities have centered on the Agency for Health Care Policy and Research (AHCPR), which was mandated in 1989 legislation to develop guidelines for common conditions and procedures. Since then, AHCPR has published more than a dozen guidelines.

The eventual purpose of clinical practice guidelines is to make practice consistent with the best evidence available. The credibility of the recommendations and the process used to develop them are likely to influence their acceptance by clinicians, patients, and the public whose behavior the guidelines are intended to influence. Guidelines formulated by AHCPR and other government agencies may be handicapped, however. A recent survey of internists suggested that physicians rank most highly guidelines developed by physician societies, followed by those developed by the National Institutes of Health, the U.S. Preventive Services Task Force, and, last, AHCPR.[1] A consortium of physician societies funded by AHCPR, as exemplified by the one which developed the otitis media with effusion guideline, thus promises to enhance the credibility and acceptance of the resulting guidelines.

The process by which guidelines are developed also might influence their adoption and use.[2] This process affects the validity of the recommendations that result and their credibility to clinicians and the public. Guideline development includes the following major activities: selection of guideline topic, task allocation of panel responsibilities, panel composition, development and evaluation of evidence, and development of conclusions and recommendations. Development of medical review and quality assessment measures and research

TABLE 1. Guideline Development Activities

Selection of Guideline Topic
>   1. Defining the guideline focus, its scope and limits
>   2. Identifying the important issues relevant to the guideline

Task Allocation, Panel Responsibilities, and Panel Constitution
>   3. Determining panel responsibilities and organization
>   4. Choosing panelists

Development and Evaluation of Evidence
>   5. Determining the rules for weighing evidence and reaching conclusions, particularly with less than adequate evidence
>   6. Selecting and evaluating the relevant literature
>   7. Evaluating the quality of the medical literature
>   8. Conducting meta-analyses and developing strategies to incorporate information not amenable to meta-analysis
>   9. Conducting economic evaluations

Development of Conclusions and Recommendations
>   10. Reaching consensus on individual findings and drafting recommendations
>   11. Synthesizing the evolved body of knowledge into a coherent guideline
>   12. Piloting the guideline and obtaining adequate scientific, clinical, and consumer input into the review of the provisional guideline

Development of Medical Review, Quality Assessment Measures
Application of Research Recommendations

---

recommendations are additional potential guideline-related activities (see table 1). In advising AHCPR, the Institute of Medicine (IOM) ranked validity as the most critical attribute of practice guidelines and stressed the importance of the credibility and accountability of the guideline development process.[3] IOM specifically recommended that feedback from guideline panels be used to examine and improve the process.

To inform guideline development as it continues to evolve at AHCPR and elsewhere, this paper analyzes the development process for the AHCPR guideline *Otitis Media with Effusion in Young Children*[4] from the perspective of two of its panel members.

Selection of Guideline Topic

Congress, in establishing AHCPR (Public Law 101-239), specified factors to be considered in setting priorities for guidelines: potential benefit for a significant number of people, reduction of clinically significant variations in services used, reduction of variations in outcomes, and the needs of the Medicare program. Reauthorizing legislation in 1992 (Public Law 102-410) added costly conditions or treatments with significant variation and likely inappropriate use. Since 1993, AHCPR has extensively solicited advice on new topics, for example, through the *Federal Register*.[5] The actual selection of guideline topics within this context has remained an internal function of agency staff.

Otitis media fit federal priorities: its prevalence among children is high; widespread variations in practice exist; questions surround the use of certain therapies; and the cost of care is high, exceeding $1 billion for ambulatory visits by young children in 1990–91.[6] Otitis media is the most frequent primary diagnosis at U.S. office visits to physicians by children younger than age fifteen;[7] a large majority of children before age six experience at least one episode of otitis media. It was not clear until the guideline development process got under way whether otitis media also fulfilled another important criteria[8]—that sufficient evidence exists on which to base recommendations.

The development of initial guidelines, when AHCPR was new and mandated to produce three within the first year, was staffed internally. When the otitis media guideline development process was begun in 1991, after identifying a general clinical condition as a priority, the agency solicited competitive proposals and contracted with an organization or consortium of organizations to produce a guideline. AHCPR then expected panels early in their deliberations to narrow their focus to a specific set of clinical issues.

AHCPR contracted with a consortium headed by the American Academy of Pediatrics that also included the American Academy of Family Physicians and the American Academy of Otolaryngology—Head and Neck Surgery to develop a guideline on otitis media. At the first meeting, the otitis media panel chair and staff directed the panel to narrow the range of issues to be addressed. The panel identified acute otitis media, recurrent otitis media, and otitis media with effusion (often a late sequela of acute and recurrent otitis) as the three major possible topics. These three conditions can be viewed as a continuum of disease. The panel debated whether an initial guideline should address the initial acute phase of illness or its late manifestations.

Acute otitis media is the most common clinical problem resulting in visits to pediatricians and family physicians in the United States and is responsible for a large portion of all antibiotic use among children. If the panel had chosen acute otitis as its focus, issues it would have addressed include the clinical criteria for diagnosis (there is no widely accepted definition of the condition), the value of antibiotics (several placebo-controlled trials have questioned the need for antibiotics in all patients), choice of antibiotics (although antibiotics costing $3–$6 per course are effective, preparations costing $50–$70 per course are commonly used), the proper duration of antibiotic treatment (2, 3, 5, 7, and 10 days have all been demonstrated to be effective), and the value and timing of various approaches to clinical follow-up.

Otitis media with effusion (OME), by contrast, is a sequela in about 20 percent of cases of acute otitis media and also develops spontaneously. OME is usually asymptomatic. Controversial issues related to the care of OME include the need for any treatment; the value of specific treatments, including antibiotics, tympanostomy tubes, adenoidectomy, and tonsillectomy; and the value of diagnostic measures in guiding treatment, including hearing assessment. Controversy exists regarding the relationship of OME to language development in young children. Controversy exists regarding the value of school and other screening programs and the relationship of OME to learning in older children.

For both acute otitis and OME, the development of rational clinical guidelines would be helpful to primary care clinicians. The research focus and clinical expertise of the already selected panel members were concentrated on OME (see Panel Composition). Although the controversies related to acute otitis media have their greatest impact on the practices of family physicians and general pediatricians, the more surgically oriented aspects of OME issues and hearing assessment are of substantial consequence to otolaryngologists and audiologists. For acute otitis, the impact of a guideline on health care costs would be through alteration in a large number of "little ticket" items involved in repeat office visits to general pediatricians and family physicians and in products of the pharmaceutical industry. By contrast, recommendations related to OME would concern "big ticket" surgical procedures that are a major source of income to otolaryngologists and could potentially increase that of audiologists.

The panel chose to focus on OME. At its second meeting it further narrowed its focus to OME in children one to three years old. In this particular case, it is unclear to what extent the importance and potential impact of the clinical issues, the overall composition of the already established panel, and the individual professional interests of panelists contributed to the choice of guideline focus. It is clearly preferable to have the guideline topic defined before an ad hoc panel is selected. More recently, AHCPR and its contractors have focused the topic before panels are chosen.

In contrast to the AHCPR process, the National Institutes of Health (NIH), with its Office of Medical Application of Research's coordination, identifies general topics to be the subjects of its consensus conferences. A planning committee is then constituted. This committee, composed of content and methods experts as well as key professional-society representatives, narrows the scope of the clinical area to be addressed and frames the consensus panel's work by composing a set of carefully worked questions for it to address.

The selection of topics for guideline development could be made through the following mechanisms: 1) the staff of the funding organization, 2) an advisory body, 3) a competitive peer review committee with the applicant required to justify the choice. Any of these could be based on expert opinion and/or data, such as indicators of importance (prevalence and cost), practice variability, availability of evidence upon which to base a guideline, and clinical importance of the topic and anticipated magnitude of impact of a guideline. A hybrid approach involving the strengths of these alternative mechanisms might be best.

Task Allocation and Panel Responsibilities

Not all of the guideline development activities need be performed by a single panel. Several functions (see table 1), such as defining the guideline focus and determining rules for weighing evidence, might best be carried out by the sponsoring organization prior to the appointing of a panel. Others, such as conducting meta-analyses, might be carried out by consultants or staff. The essential functions of the core panel are to ensure that the appropriate breadth of scientific and clinical information has been considered and that the synthesis of information has been conducted rationally and is incorporated into the final guideline statement.

Of the nineteen members of the OME guideline panel, very few had expertise in research methods, including statistics and epidemiology. This situation made review of studies and formulation of valid recommendations difficult. At an early meeting the panel was asked to develop a strategy for identifying relevant studies and criteria for including and excluding certain studies. At the fourth meeting, subgroups for specific topics, such as antibiotics or surgical interventions, reviewed the research design of each study to determine whether or not it should be included in meta-analyses. Each member's understanding of the literature also underlay voting on recommendations. The panel's methodologist was well versed in critical analysis and had worked with other guideline panels, but his skills could not compensate at key points in the process for the panel's methods weakness.

In response to the need for methods expertise, one approach is to limit panel membership to methods experts, including clinicians with training in research design. The U.S. Preventive Services Task Force used a variant of this approach. Its standing committee consisted of generalist physicians and some methods experts, although an earlier committee also included nursing and economic expertise. Content specialists served in a consultant role to present information and review drafts. This approach is at least partly intended to temper the influence of specialists attuned to the use of their own field's tools. The recommendations of the task force are well known for their rigor. Even the most sensitive physicians, however, may not perceive matters of great import to patients or to other health professionals.

An alternative is to establish a two-stage process. A large panel would select the issues to be considered in developing a guideline for a predetermined topic. A small group with methods and clinical expertise then would identify and review studies. This group could present tabulations of the evidence to the large, broader panel. The larger panel would then deliberate and formulate recommendations for the guideline. The small group would include content specialists and serve as members of, or consultants to, the larger panel. This approach retains the advantages of the multidisciplinary panel, while incorporating technical expertise into the review and tabulation of evidence.

Panel Composition

The legislation establishing AHCPR stipulated that guideline panels should be composed of "appropriately qualified experts," including physicians with appropriate expertise and from different practice settings, and health care consumers. Reauthorization language in 1992 stated that clinicians whose incomes might be affected by the guideline should not be overly represented, but did not set specific limits. The 1992 law also required that at least one participant have expertise in epidemiology and the clinical topic and at least one have expertise in health services research or health economics and the clinical topic.

For the otitis media guideline, the contractor was responsible for selecting panel members, subject to AHCPR's approval. The consortium initially proposed a fifteen-person panel, based on expertise, geography, ethnicity, and gender. After the first meeting, two were replaced because of conflicts of interest related to pharmaceutical funding. After a *Federal Register* notice and additional solicitations, four more people were added.[9] The panel, cochaired by a pediatric otolaryngologist and a clinical epidemiologist, consisted of five otolaryngologists, three family physicians (including the cochair), two pediatricians, two nurse-practitioners, and a single infectious-disease specialist, maternal and child health nurse, audiologist, psychologist, speech-language pathologist, economist, and consumer representative. As a result of this diversity, the panel's deliberations incorporated a wide range of clinical situations and policy issues. The broad range of perspectives and expertise on the panel is a hallmark of AHCPR's process, for guideline development as well as for other activities.

The importance of panel composition is well known.[10] Panel composition might affect the topics selected for guidelines, the credibility of the guidelines to others, and the content of the guidelines recommendations. As one would expect, specialists in a given field are more likely to agree and more likely to deem procedures used in their field to be appropriate. "Balanced" panels composed of multiple specialists, such as the OME one, are intended to avoid bias for or against any one field. An alternative outcome, however, is that the various specialties trade off uncritical acceptance of each other's activities.

Although perhaps not generalizable to other panels, the contentious situation concerning the OME panel chair is noteworthy. He was chairman of a department in which a bitter controversy about the efficacy of antibiotic therapy for otitis media had split the faculty.[11] The chair had not been part of this conflict, and the matter seemed no longer to be active when the consortium and AHCPR selected the panel. When it erupted again shortly after the panel first met,[12] and was raised at the public hearing, the panel established special procedures to review the disputed studies, and the chair recused himself from all discussions of antibiotics. In addition, the contractor appointed a panel cochair. The contractor and panel expected that these measures would ensure the validity and credibility of the recommendations.

The broad composition of AHCPR's guideline panels to date has been both a strength and a weakness. Their multidisciplinary composition brings a wide range of perspectives and issues to panel deliberations and is likely to improve the eventual acceptance and implementation of a guideline. It also promotes a philosophy of inclusion, especially for consumers and nonphysician health professionals. As already discussed, the major deficiency is the need for additional technical expertise to evaluate the validity of studies and their results.

Using another model, the U.S. Preventive Services Task Force has relied on a core committee of generalist physicians from family practice, internal medicine, pediatrics, and obstetrics-gynecology, supplemented by content experts who serve on the panel during consideration of certain topics.[13] This approach allows the core group to gain experience with the guideline process and assessment methods but entails its own orientation or bias, in this case in favor of primary care.

As a response to these issues, other organizations have taken different approaches to structuring guideline panels. The NIH Consensus Conference planning committees identify potential panelists and organizations to be consulted. Thereafter, the panels are constituted by NIH staff. Specialty societies have various approaches to staffing guideline development. These often include a standing committee to overview their activity, and subcommittees constituted for specific guidelines.

Panels increasingly have recognized the importance of methodological expertise. The U.S. Preventive Services Task Force included an epidemiologist and a decision analyst. Following an evaluation of the National Institutes of Health Consensus Development Program, NIH has included two methodologists, such as an epidemiologist and a biostatistician, on each of its panels.[14]

A related issue is that no formal mechanism exists to monitor and revise the OME guideline. The ad hoc nature of the OME panel, its sponsorship, and its membership preclude an orderly and regular process of evaluating new evidence or updating the guideline. AHCPR is moving to standing panels appointed for five years. This will create a structure within which regular review and updating of guidelines becomes feasible.

Development and Evaluation of Evidence

AHCPR panels have typically used evidence-based methods to produce guidelines.[15] A panel identifies and synthesizes the literature, holds public hearings, and combines evidence and expert opinion to produce recommendations. The first four meetings of the OME panel were devoted to instruction in meta-analysis and guideline development methods, defining the topic of interest, identifying relevant literature, hearing public testimony, and weighing the quality of the literature. Coached by the methodologist, the OME panel used some of the explicit methods of guideline development formulated by David Eddy. Where the literature permitted, the methodologist performed quantitative meta-analyses to derive the likely health benefits and harms of interventions. Following finalization of recommendations at the last panel meeting, staff prepared algorithms and distributed them for comment.

Once the panel chose OME as its topic, it set about identifying the major treatment options and issues involved for literature review and meta-analysis. The abstraction of articles for the literature review was conducted by fellows and graduate students at the panel chairman's department. The methodologist was at a distant location. Although most panelists had little involvement in the search activity for practical reasons, they did oversee the process. For example, in at least one area—the impact of OME on speech and language development—several panelists professionally involved in the area felt that a considerable body of literature had been missed, and the panel formed a subcommittee to extend the literature review and weigh the evidence in this area.

The department conducting the literature review had little experience in formal review or quantitative meta-analysis. Much of the abstracted material, especially about study design, was inaccurate. Since the panel subgroups used these abstracts to select or eliminate studies for further analysis, these errors had the potential to undermine the validity of the selections made. In practice, it is likely that errors with the potential to affect the recommendations were corrected. Some of the panel subgroups, including the one on surgical interventions, rechecked the design of each study; the methodologist re-abstracted all antibiotics studies and others considered critical to the recommendations; and a highly accurate abstractor reabstracted some studies.

Panelists divided into subcommittees to assess the quality of articles related to diagnostic, therapeutic, and outcomes issues. The importance of making this evaluation based on an assessment of methods while blinded to the results was presented by the panel methodologist. Panelists were observed, however, to include and even start their evaluations of an article by reviewing its results and conclusion.

The importance of having the literature review and abstracting done by experienced people or under the close supervision of an experienced person has been recognized, as has the use of meta-analysis to weigh evidence. Perhaps not as widely appreciated, structuring a guideline within an algorithm framework may help identify and clarify issues, especially those related to clinical decisions and their timing, sequence, and applicability to various patient groups. In contrast to the experience of the OME panel, algorithm development should start early, with restructuring of the guideline algorithm(s) as the panel clarifies its findings and recommendations.

The abstraction of the literature, composition of meta-analyses, and algorithm construction are technical activities requiring specific expertise and involving teams who gain experience from working together. Staffing these tasks for multiple guideline panels with a permanent team might yield improvements in both quality and efficiency while decreasing the time required.

Panel process and time allocation are also important determinants of the quality of a guideline. Once initial guideline components and recommendations have been considered, commonly a second set of issues and decisions is formulated for which the evaluation of evidence also is indicated. For the OME guideline, once the panel established the importance of testing hearing, the secondary issue of determining the threshold hearing level for clinical decisions became apparent. Because of a lack of time, the panel based the crucial decision of the level requiring intervention on the expert opinion of those few panelists professionally most involved with testing. Without considering evidence, a threshold level of 20 dB was chosen as indicating the need for tympanostomy tube insertion; a 30 dB threshold level would have decreased by over 50 percent the number of children annually who would have ear tubes indicated.[16] Of note, a 30 dB level or worse is the level commonly used to indicate intervention with children with permanent hearing loss. Thus, this opinion translates into the indication for several hundred thousand tympanostomy tube insertions at a cost of up to a billion dollars a year. Clearly, time and financial support for guideline development must be realistic, but they must also be flexible enough to allow crucial unanticipated issues identified late in the process to be resolved adequately.

Guidelines of AHCPR and other organizations have not typically included economic analysis. The OME guideline contained only a brief and general analysis of the cost implications of its recommendations. The paucity of administrative data on OME separate from otitis media in general handicapped the cost analysis. The lack of a more thorough cost analysis is especially striking, however, because the cost implications of tympanostomy tubes underlay at least some panelists' support of a guideline on OME instead of the other potential topics, extensive resources went to a subcontractor for cost analysis, and of the published AHCPR guidelines, only the OME panel has included an economist.

Change at AHCPR is already under way in this area. Perhaps in response to legislative interest, AHCPR has contracted for cost analyses of several guidelines to be developed during the coming year. Cost-effectiveness analysis is being incorporated into the development of at least one guideline. Both cost-effectiveness analysis and budgetary or cost analysis have important complementary roles to play in clinical guidelines. Cost-effectiveness analysis, which compares the costs and health effects of alternative strategies for managing a condition, can inform the panel about the implications of specific interventions. Analysis of the total cost implications of a guideline for society and perhaps for certain payers addresses the overall affordability of the guideline recommendations.

Development of Conclusions and Recommendations

The role of panel opinion, scientific evidence in determining recommendations, and the methods to be used in decision making to ensure such ownership all became issues for the OME panel.

The OME panel limited its consideration of outcomes to those for which it had, or thought the literature would provide, objective measures. In so doing, it omitted consideration of most behavioral or symptom-related issues, including ones that motivate parents to bring their children for care and thus often are given priority by clinicians in determining the care they provide. Specifically, the panel heard, but did not consider further, anecdotal evidence of chronically unhappy and irritable children whose behavior improved dramatically following insertion of tympanostomy tubes. Ironically, although it limited itself to considering only outcomes for which objective measures were reported in the literature, for most of the questions that the panel wished to address, it subsequently found the quality of the available evidence to be poor. Consequently, most of the conclusions are based substantially upon panelists' opinion.

In particular, adequate scientific evidence was found missing in two crucial areas. First, there is little basis upon which to assess the importance of OME to long-term outcomes, including language development and school performance. Since most OME is asymptomatic, this issue is central to determining the need for *any* intervention. There also was virtually no evidence regarding the presence or importance of symptoms or their effect on either the child's or the family's quality of life. As a result, the panel ignored quality-of-life issues in reaching its conclusions.

Second, the panel recommends hearing testing of all children with three months of documented effusion. This is one of the major recommendations likely to change routine practice and is essential to the assessment and treatment approach put forward by the panel. Although it acknowledges that such testing might be difficult to obtain in some rural areas, it neither provides alternatives nor discusses the implications of the lack of availability of such testing for its recommendations. In part, this omission is based on the opinion of some panelists that the technology is available and therefore its lack in some communities is simply a local deficiency that must be resolved. Unfortunately, this view does not take into account the complex issues involved in creating and maintaining specialty medical services in some rural and urban areas.

The OME panel decision-making process was problematic. Tabulations of benefits and harms of each considered intervention were available only on overhead transparencies and only at the final meeting during which the panel voted on the guideline recommendations. Tabulations were not available to individual panel members until after drafts of the guideline text had been circulated to the panel for review. This situation made it difficult for members to assess the accuracy and tone of the final recommendations.

The panel resolved controversies by majority vote. Most of the panel recommendations were voted on during a few hours of two afternoons of panel meetings. This occurred under time pressure and with inadequate discussion. More time for discussion might have allowed panelists to identify the sources of their differences and develop objective means of narrowing them. Instead, such vote-derived "consensus" often involved a choice between two opposing positions strongly held by a few members of the panel, with other panelists relying on the reports of subcommittees and the oral persuasiveness of position advocates.

The marked difference in positions held by various members of the panel and the lack of true resolution of these differences are reflected in the final guideline documents. For example, given the limited evidence of the efficacy of antibiotics, in the chapter on drug treatments the panel presents antibiotics as an option rather than a recommendation; in the chapter on surgical treatments and in the algorithm, however, it recommends that antibiotics be given to all children not receiving ear tubes by three months. The influence of those panelists convinced that OME has significant long-term impact is reflected in statements which overinterpret nonsignificant study results, such as "Some cohort studies reported greater variance within groups than between groups on standardized measures of speech or language, suggesting a complex relationship between developmental delays and otitis media with effusion." In contrast, a more prudent opinion is reflected in conclusions such as, "The Panel found that rigorous, methodologically sound research does not adequately support or refute the theory that untreated otitis media with effusion results in speech/language delays or deficits."

Ownership of the OME guideline became a concern. Throughout most of the guideline development process, the consortium and AHCPR officials clearly stated that responsibility for, and control over, the guideline's content rested with the panel. Largely because identification of the topic and problems with abstracting consumed many months early in the OME panel's life, the consortium and AHCPR faced great time pressure at the end of the project. Only the last two meetings involved discussion of the issues and alternatives available to the panel in defining guideline recommendations. Given the early delay, much of the OME panel's later interaction about the content and tone of the recommendations occurred by correspondence after all the scheduled and budgeted meetings had been held.

The guideline adopted by the panel was circulated for peer review to more than 100 individuals and organizations. The consortium, cochairs, and AHCPR staff met to incorporate reviewers' comments and circulated some of the changes back to the panel. At some time after the final meeting and some months before publication, ownership of the guideline seemed to shift from the panel to the consortium sponsors and AHCPR. A professional writer attended several panel meetings and prepared the guideline text, most of which occurred after the final meeting. A mail ballot on certain unresolved and protested issues was circulated to the panel after its last meeting. Upon review of the circulated draft, some panel members objected to other parts of the guideline in both content and tone; these objections, however, were not shared with other panelists or addressed. The guideline itself states that a technical report[17] includes a minority comment, but it was not circulated to the entire panel. The panel was not asked to sign off on the final guideline text.

Although projects and committees inevitably face unforeseen delays and pressing deadlines, groups developing guidelines should consider procedures, used by two other organizations, related to obtaining external review and maintaining panel authority. The U.S. Preventive Services Task Force purposefully sought dissenting views during its review process. It held formal votes on all points, and if the vote was close, the dissenting minority was asked to present new evidence for further discussion. The Institute of Medicine also selects and staffs committees, but IOM committees then maintain authority over their final reports. Individual committee members must provide written approval of the final text or may submit a dissenting statement to be included.

Based on the OME panel's experience, the initial change to the panel should specify the role of panel opinion and scientific evidence in determining recommendations, the methods to be used in decision making and resolving controversies, the final ownership of the guideline, and the methods to be used to ensure such ownership. For standing panels, refinement of these issues over time might provide an enduring advance for the field.

Development of Medical Review and Quality Assessment Measures

Following the completion of the guideline and the guideline's release, the sponsors reconvened the OME panel to develop medical-review criteria and performance standards. These were included in phase 2 of the contractor's scope of work. The panel voiced considerable concern with the concept of developing performance standards, for fear that they might be used inappropriately for utilization review by managed care companies. It did issue measures that it qualified as being appropriate for quality improvement activities based on aggregate data but not for individual case review.

Staff of the consortium contracted to develop the guideline developed preliminary review criteria and pilot-tested them in several practices. This pilot activity and subsequent panel discussion confirmed a number of logical inconsistencies and ambiguities in the original OME guideline recommendations, particularly problems related to the implementation of the recommendations over a series of visits during the course of an episode of OME. For example, although a hearing test is an option before three months of persistent effusion, it is recommended at three months. A hearing test also is recommended before a decision to insert tympanostomy tubes is made. The clinician, however, acting within the recommendations, might not insert tympanostomy tubes until six months. In this circumstance, the three-month hearing test would have no impact on clinical decision making at three months and would not be timely for use in decision making at six months. The panel had not intended that repeated testing be done in such cases. Although the panel finessed this issue in developing its review criteria, it was troubled by the inconsistency of its original guideline statement. If the panel had been charged with developing the medical-review criteria as part of its core guideline development process, this inconsistency would have been corrected. The development of a guideline algorithm is closely related to the development of review criteria, and these might best be done together during the process of weighing evidence and making recommendations. This experience also highlights the value of piloting guideline recommendations, algorithms, and medical-review criteria with feedback to the panel before the guideline is finalized.

Translating Research Recommendations into Program Priorities

A major contribution of the guideline development process is the systematic identification of gaps in existing knowledge. The guideline process can indicate whether the gap is important or unimportant for clinical and public policy, and brings it to the immediate attention of the panel and sponsoring organizations. Important deficiencies should feed directly into priorities for funding relevant research by government agencies, such as AHCPR, the National Institutes of Health, and the Centers for Disease Control and Prevention; professional societies; and health-related foundations. Currently no formal mechanism for this exists.

Conclusion

Guideline development is complex and potentially subject to numerous problems. The examination of the process undertaken by the OME panel provides guidance for improving guideline development processes. AHCPR, professional societies, and others promoting evidence-based practice face the continuing challenge of building on past experience to improve the validity and credibility of future guidelines.

NOTES

1. S. R. Tunis et al., "Internists' Attitudes about Clinical Practice Guidelines," *Annals of Internal Medicine* 120 (1994): 956–63.

2. J. M. Grimshaw and I. T. Russell, "Effect of Clinical Guidelines on Medical

Practice: A Systematic Review of Rigorous Evaluations," *Lancet* 342 (1993): 1317–33; U.S. Congress, Office of Technology Assessment, *Identifying Health Technologies That Work: Searching for Evidence* (Washington, D. C.: U.S. Government Printing Office, 1994).

    3. Institute of Medicine, *Clinical Practice Guidelines: Directions for a New Program* (Washington, D. C.: National Academy Press, 1990).

    4. S. E. Stool et al., *Otitis Media with Effusion in Young Children: Clinical Practice Guidelines*, No. 12, AHCPR Publication No. 94-0622, Rockville, Md.: Agency for Health Care Policy and Research, Public Health Services, U.S. Department of Health and Human Services AHCPR Publication No. 94-0622, 1994.

    5. U.S. Congress, Office of Technology Assessment, *Identifying Health Technologies That Work*.

    6. S. E. Stool et al., *Otitis Media with Effusion*.

    7. S. M. Shappert, "Office Visits for Otitis Media: United States, 1975–90," in *Advance Data from Vital and Health Statistics of the Centers for Disease Control/National Center for Health Statistics* (Washington, D. C.: U.S. Department of Health and Human Services, 1992).

    8. P. M. Wortman, A. Vinokur, and L. Sechrest, "Do Consensus Conferences Work? A Process Evaluation of the NIH Consensus Development Program," *J Health Politics, Policy, and Law* 13 (1988): 469–98.

    9. S. E. Stool et al., *Otitis Media with Effusion*.

    10. P. M. Wortman, A. Vinokur, and L. Sechrest, "Do Consensus Conferences Work?"; R. Grol, "Development of Guidelines for General Practice Care," *Br J Gen Prac* 43 (1993): 146–51; L. L. Leape et al., "Group Judgments of Appropriateness: The Effect of Panel Composition," *Quality Assurance in Health Care* 4 (1992): 151–9.

    11. D. Rennie, "The Cantekin Affair," *JAMA* 266, no. 23 (1991): 3333–7.

    12. E. I. Cantekin, T. W. McGuire, and T. L. Griffith, "Antimicrobial Therapy for Otitis Media with Effusion," *JAMA* 266 (1991): 3309–17.

    13. S. H. Woolf and H. C. J. Sox, "The Expert Panel on Preventive Services: Continuing the Work of the U.S. Preventive Services Task Force," *Am J Prev Med* 7 (1991): 326–30.

    14. P. M. Workman, A. Vinokur, and L. Sechrest, "Do Consensus Conferences Work?"

    15. S. H. Woolf and H. C. J. Sox, "The Expert Panel on Preventive Services."

    16. L. Culpepper and J. Froom, "Otitis Media with Effusion in Young Children: Treatment in Search of a Problem." *J Amer Board of Family Practice* 8, no. 4 (1995): 1–12.

    17. S. E. Stool et al., *Otitis Media with Effusion in Young Children: Guideline Technical Report*, No. 12, AHCPR Publication No. 95-0621 (Rockville, Md.: Agency for Health Care Policy and Research, Public Health Services, U.S. Department of Health and Human Services, 1995).

Gert Jan van der Wilt and Peter F. de Vries Robbé

The Quest for the Trial to End All Trials

Introduction

"In fact, technology assessors are strongly interested in improving quality of care, as shown in their professional literature. They have not, however, found fully satisfactory pathways to this goal."[1]

In the above statement, David Banta clearly expresses what he thinks is the major rationale and justification of medical technology assessment: the desire to improve the quality of medical care. He also observes that medical technology assessment has not fully lived up to this objective. In the present chapter we wish to pursue this inadequacy in a particular case: studies that have been carried out in the field of glue ear (otitis media with effusion, OME) and its medical management.

Glue ear is a common condition among children, many of whom receive medical treatment. In the United States, the prevalence rate of ventilation tubes (VTs) was estimated to be 13 per 1,000 children aged younger than eighteen years in 1988.[2] The question is whether, and in which cases, medical treatment is necessary. In spite of the fact that many clinical trials have been conducted in this area, many clinicians feel that this issue has as yet not been satisfactorily resolved.[3] The purpose of this chapter is to reflect on the possible causes of the current predicament and to discuss possibilities for amelioration. The chapter will summarize what is known about the natural history and treatment of glue ear, how it has been treated in the past and how it is currently treated. The nature of the controversies that have persisted to this day will be analyzed, and it will be argued that it is important to distinguish between disagreements over the credibility of the data and disagreements over the relevance of the data.

Epidemiology and Natural History of Glue Ear

Glue ear is a condition characterized by the presence of fluid (effusion) in the middle-ear cavity without any signs or symptoms of ear infection (such as bulging eardrum usually accompanied by pain, or perforated eardrum often with drainage of purulent material).[4] If pain is present with the condition, it is usually intermittent and mild.[5] Glue ear may be identified following an acute episode of otitis media or following a routine screening test for hearing (such as the Ewing test). Symptoms may include discomfort or behavior changes.[6]

Glue ear is the most common cause of hearing impairment and most common reason for elective surgery in children; 75–95 percent of all children have had at least one episode of otitis media by the age of six.[7] Glue ear resolves spontaneously in the majority of children although recurrence is common. Most episodes are of short duration: around 50 percent of affected ears resolve spontaneously after three months and only 5 percent of children will have glue ear for a period of a year or more. The hearing loss associated with OME usually is in the range of 15–35 dB, and typically probably ca. 25 dB. A normal hearing threshold is ca. 15dB; hence, in a child with bilateral effusion in the middle ear, this hearing threshold will usually be between 25 and 40dB.[8] Such a hearing loss means that a child may miss softer speech sounds.

A major question is whether such a hearing loss is potentially developmentally compromising. The results of the Greater Boston Otitis Media Study Group indicate that at the age of seven, children who experience more than 130 days with middle-ear effusion during their first three years of life are measurably different from their peers who experience less than 30 days with middle-ear effusion during these years. "Measurably different" here means, among other things, the difference between an average IQ of 117 and an average IQ of 109.[9] In the Dunedin study, a positive correlation was also found between episodes of OME during childhood and later-life development.[10] In many other studies, however, no such correlation could be found.[11]

Treatment of Glue Ear, 1860–1960

A beautiful historic overview of the treatment of glue ear can be found in Black.[12] Briefly, during the 1860s, Adam Politzer used tympanostomy tubes (grommets) in the treatment of glue ear. The rationale for tubes was the attempt to remove secretion from the middle ear by delaying healing of the incised tympanic membrane or making a permanent opening. By 1890, this mode of treatment was largely abandoned, partly because of the high complication rate (postmyringotomy middle-ear infection). Instead, glue ear was treated by adeno-tonsillectomy. From the 1920s to the 1950s, the use of ionizing radiation (instead of surgical removal) to shrink nasopharyngeal lymphoid tissue became widely adopted as a treatment for glue ear. Black writes that the "reason for abandonment of radiation is not made explicit in the literature—a combination of concern about its ineffectiveness at curing deafness, possible long term harmful effects, and the increasing commitment to surgical and other therapies may all have contributed." Among the other therapies were allergy control and vaccination. In 1954, Armstrong reintroduced the insertion of ventilating tubes for treatment of glue ear. Probably the availability of chemotherapy to treat postoperative infections has contributed to this newly gained wider acceptance. Also, changes in the design enabled the tubes to remain in place longer. Since the 1960s, myringotomy, tube insertion, adenoidectomy, and tonsillectomy have been used in various combinations in the treatment of glue ear. Since that time, the overall number of operations for glue ear has increased considerably.[13] As possible reasons for this increase, Black[14] mentions: (1) the widespread introduction of audiometry, which resulted in increased detection of glue ear, (2) greater recognition of the presence of fluid in the middle ear by general practitioners, (3) the availability of more otolaryngologists, (4) the availability of antibiotics to treat postoperative infections, (5) the need of surgeons to fill the vacuum caused by the decline in the number of adenotonsillectomies for other indications, and (6) the fact that glue ear provides parents with a medical explanation for their children's poor school performance.

Current Treatment of Glue Ear

Current treatment patterns of glue ear have been reported in several studies, revealing considerable geographic variation. Black[15] found up to sevenfold differences in surgical rates for glue ear between districts in the UK. Wide disparities in the management of glue ear among ENT consultants in the United Kingdom have also been documented by Smith et al.[16] and by Smith and Maw.[17] In an Australian study also documenting such variation, the authors state that they "found no evidence that the National Health and Medical Research Council Tonsillectomy and Adenoidectomy Guidelines (first published in 1982) have been effective in influencing clinical practice."[18] Concern about inappropriate treatment has given rise to appropriateness research: comparing medical practice with a norm for appropriate medical management. Spilseth[19] concludes that among thirty-eight children who had received tubes for glue ear, twenty were appropriate indications for tube insertion. A much larger study was recently conducted in the United States, scrutinizing the appropriateness recommendations that 6,611 children receive tympanostomy tubes.[20] Criteria for appropriateness were developed by an expert panel, consisting of five pediatricians and four otolaryngologists, using a two-round Delphi method. In the study, 42 percent of the proposals were appropriate,

35 percent equivocal, and 23 percent inappropriate. "Appropriate tube placements" were defined as those for which the expected health benefits exceeded the expected negative health consequences by a sufficiently wide margin that the procedure was worth doing; explicit considerations of financial costs were excluded. Criteria for assessing appropriateness included otoscopic findings, results of hearing tests, age, and one or more courses of antibiotics. In view of the low degree of agreement on the optimal management of glue ear, it is not surprising that the conclusions of this appropriateness study were challenged, too. The criteria for appropriateness were considered far too stringent.[21]

Studies of Treatment Effects

Ventilation Tubes

Several studies have shown that insertion of ventilation tubes in children with OME restores the pre-effusion level of hearing acuity.[22] As long as the tubes remain in place, hearing level will be usually normal. The average "tube-survival period" is ca. six to twelve months. Because of the high rate of spontaneous resolution, however, the difference between treated and not-treated usually declines with time. Most studies show a benefit three months after the intervention (defined as a mean decrease in hearing threshold of 6–12 dB), which has disappeared twelve months after the intervention.[23]

In a study by Lildholdt,[24] the hearing improvement resulting from tube insertion was of much shorter duration. It was observed only up to three weeks postoperatively. Lildholdt concludes that tube insertion may be indicated because of the hearing loss associated with OME but that it should be borne in mind that it involves a high risk of complications:

- Insertion of VTs usually takes place under general anesthesia; the probability of adverse events as the result of general anesthesia is low but not negligible.
- Scarring of the tympanic membrane (in ca. 50 percent of the cases); in a study by Tos and Stangerup,[25] it was found that this most commonly observed side effect resulted in a hearing impairment of less than 0.5 dB, which is inconsequential and cannot serve as an argument against the use of VTs.
- Recurrent infection around the tube (25 percent or more).
- Permanent perforation (3 percent).
- Cholesteatoma: a skin growth that occurs in the middle ear typically caused by repeated infections of this area. Over time, it can take the form of a cyst, destroying the tissues and structures of the middle ear.

Apart from the effects of tube insertion on effusion and hearing acuity, indications exist that tube insertion has a favorable effect on child behavior. In a study conducted by Manders and Tyberghein,[26] parents of children who had had tubes inserted for OME were asked about their experience. Fifty-five percent of the parents noticed some kind of change in behavior after surgery ("became more open," "is happier since," "is more pleasant"). All parents in this study were satisfied about having the tube placement done for of better hearing (50 percent), improved general health (28 percent), or both (21 percent). Sixty-one percent of the parents reported improvement in their child's comprehension, though positive changes in speech and language were scarcely reported. Parents observed that their children were responding more quickly to questions, were more alert to sounds, joined more in conversations, etc.

Not all children with OME stand to benefit equally from VTs. The heterogeneity of the population of children with glue ear is considerable. At one extreme, there is the "OME-prone child": a child who has the condition six or more times before the age of six or whose initial episode of otitis media was due to pneumococcus and occurred before the age of one.[27] At the other extreme, there is the child with a short-lasting, spontaneously resolving episode of OME that produces such weak symptoms that it passes by unrecognized. Such cases may be detected through screening programs for hearing disorders in children, such as the Ewing screening. This screening modality was set up for the early identification of children with sensorineural hearing loss, not children with conductive hearing losses, as in the case of OME. The otitis-prone child will benefit much more from treatment with tube insertion than the child with mild OME. It is, however, at present not possible to predict very well whether, and by how much, a child with OME will benefit from treatment.[28]

Alternative Modes of Treatment

Many children with OME are treated with an antihistamine decongestant. There is good evidence, however, that such treatment is totally ineffective.[29] Another common treatment modality is antibiotics. In a study conducted by Mandel et al., 29 percent of the children with OME and treated with amoxicillin were OME-free after a period of four weeks. In children who received a placebo, this figure was 14 percent ($p<0.001$). There were no statistically significant differences between the groups in the mean hearing thresholds or in the amount of improvement in hearing acuity. As side effects of the antibiotic, parents reported mild diarrhea and a rash (both in 3 out of 160). Cautiously, the authors conclude that "amoxicillin treatment increases to some extent the likelihood of resolution."[30]

With respect to adenoidectomy, the situation is more complicated. A number of trials have been conducted that failed to show any effect of adenoidectomy.[31] The study by Fiellau-Nikolajsen was a randomized controlled trial involving forty-two three-year-old children with OME that had persisted for at least six months; it failed to reveal any differenece in middle-ear status between the experimental group (adenoidectomy and myringotomy) and the control group (myringotomy alone). The authors admit that the trial was of limited size, but argue that this was ethically appropriate since a therapeutic method was tested "to which the great majority of experts attribute a definite value." They continue by stating that their results "pave the way for broadly designed, multi-centre studies."

Such a study was conducted by Bulman et al.[32] Ironically, the authors hoped that the results of this trial would justify withholding adenoidectomy in the routine surgical treatment of children with deafness due to exudative otitis media, but this aim has not been achieved.[33] Instead, the authors had to conclude that "adenoidectomy seems to play a significant role in the medium term prophylaxis of hearing loss due to exudative otitis media." In a later study,[34] Gates et al. recommend that in children with persistent OME unresponsive to treatment with antibiotics and decongestants during a sixty-day period, adenoidectomy is the treatment of choice, accompanied by myringotomy to remove effusion.

Discussion

We started this chapter by quoting David Banta's observation that technology assessors are strongly interested in improving quality of care but that they have not found fully satisfactory pathways to this goal. This observation seems to hold true in the case of OME and its medical management. The rationale and justification of studies in this field can only be the desire to improve the management of the condition by obtaining answers to questions such as these: Should at least some of the children with OME receive medical treatment, and if so, which treatment and why? What is the nature of the benefit that will then be produced? Clearly, however, no unequivocal answers have materialized from these studies. There is no agreement on the long-term consequences of OME during childhood, nor is there agreement on optimal treatment.

Studies of OME have been criticized for many reasons, including inadequate design giving rise to biased observations, the questionable validity and reliability of developmental tests, inadequate ascertainment of the presence of OME and of hearing loss, confounding, small sample size, nonrepresentativeness of subjects, etc.[35] We are faced with a wide variety of studies, differing in design, patient population, outcome measures, time horizon, treatment comparisons, etc. In the absence of agreed-upon standards of care, it is difficult, if not outright impossible, to assess the quality of the care that is provided in the management of OME. The considerable variation in medical practice, however, casts doubt on the quality of care and suggests that there is still considerable potential for improvement.

It is tempting to try to devise a conclusive, or "definitive,"[36] study, a trial to end all trials. But it is hard to see why a future study, however carefully designed, would not be susceptible to at least some of the criticism that has been leveled at previous studies, unless we get a better understanding of the nature of these criticisms. Apart from methodological rigor, agreement is needed on the rationale for treatment and/or the minimal difference between treated and nontreated children that is still to be considered meaningful.

Is It True? Does It Matter?

To illustrate this, take the following example: A randomized controlled trial has shown that in a specified population (defined by explicit inclusion and exclusion criteria) of children with persistent bilateral OME, insertion of ventilation tubes results in a mean decrease of the hearing threshold of 10dB at 1000 Hz, as compared to doing nothing, at six months postoperatively. The difference was statistically significant, in the sense that the probability of such a difference being due to chance alone was less than 0.05. From the result of the study the authors conclude that children who would have been eligible for the study, ought to be treated by insertion of ventilation tubes in their eardrums.

With respect to the statements that are made in the context of this study, two questions can and probably should be asked: Are they true? Do they matter? The first question raises the issue of credibility; any suspicion of bias casts doubt on the findings of the study. The second question raises the issue of relevance, as when critics argue that a mean difference of 10dB in hearing threshold is not a meaningful difference or indeed that hearing acuity is not an appropriate end point at all. Contentions that six months following the intervention is too short a period for appraisal, that inappropriate alternatives for comparison were included, that the study sample was not representative, or that the study was underpowered statistically are also of this type. The credibility of the data gathered is not so much challenged, but it is held that the relevant follow-up period has not been observed, the relevant comparisons have not been made, the relevant end point has not been measured, or the relevant patient population has not been included in the study. Similarly, to call a study underpowered means that it will not, because of its size (the number of patients that were enrolled), be capable of finding a meaningful difference between groups, if such a difference exists. Such criticisms indicate a difference of opinion as to what constitutes a meaningful difference between research groups ("a difference that makes a difference"). Claims of "nonrepresentativeness" or "limited generalizability" also address the relevance question. Patients who were selected for the study may not be representative of the wider population of patients with the relevant condition; patient selection thus renders the study itself irrelevant. Finally, we must ask, difference to whom? that is, which perspective is taken into account: the perspective of the hospital manangement, the patient, society at large?

It is not self-evident whether the value of VTs should be assessed in terms of disease-current (effusion, hearing acuity, child behavior) or in terms of disease-consequent phenomena (child development). Although it is relatively straightforward to demonstrate the disease-current benefits of the intervention, when these are the only benefits of the intervention, it is questionable whether they outweigh the risks associated with the procedure and whether the commitment of communal resources for treatment of OME is justified (limited relevance). Demonstrating disease-consequent benefits of the procedure would eliminate such doubts. In this respect, it is significant that long-term risks associated with the condition are used to argue for its potential value: "There are children in the industrial world who have linguistic deficiencies and subsequent economic and social disadvantages because they were not identified at the optimal time as having a hearing impairment. . . . Linguistic deficits result in a greater social cost than they did 50 years ago. The societal environment modifies the definition and effect of disease. Communication skills are now more valuable to the population than at any other time in history."[37]

Demonstrating the disease-consequent benefits of the procedure, however, is much more troublesome (relevance is gained at the expense of credibility). For that purpose, children suffering from chronic OME during infancy would have to be randomly allocated to an experimental group (VTs) and a control group (no treatment). The follow-up period would have to be several years to assess whether tube insertion in these children makes a meaningful difference in speech and language development. We are not saying that such research cannot be done; what we are saying is that it probably cannot be done in such a way as to leave ample opportunity for criticism on the part of those who are skeptical of surgical treatment of glue ear. As Ruben[38] observed: "The minimal amount of auditory deprivation which is necessary to result in a cognitive defect in man is not known. . . . There is no simple answer that can define, in quantitative terms, the measures of outcome of sensory deprivation, because many of the measures are qualitative, judgemental and socially defined."

Resolve Factual and Moral Uncertainties

The continuing research efforts of the past decades have been met with an unwillingness on the part of the professional community to accept the collected evidence as conclusive. We cannot demonstrate conclusively that leaving pediatric OME untreated is developmentally compromising, nor the opposite, that it is not. In such situations, it is the allocation of the burden of proof that critically determines whether we will continue to treat OME surgically or abandon this practice.[39] Do we give the benefit of the doubt to VTs, and only stop doing so when it has been established that the benefits do not outweigh the risks and costs? Or should we only insert ventilation tubes when it has been convincingly established that the benefits outweigh the risks and costs? Highly illustrative in this respect is the conclusion, reached by the Agency for Health Care Policy and Research (AHCPR) in its recent guideline for the treatment of glue ear: "Although there is insufficient evidence to prove that there are long-term deleterious effects of OME, concern about the possibility of such effects led the panel to recommend surgery, based on their expert opinion."[40]

Is there anything that we can do to alter the current situation? I would suggest that, before embarking on a new clinical trial, we should squarely face the question, What is it that we don't know (with sufficient certainty) about glue ear and its medical management and that matters? To answer that question, we should determine the rationale for treatment of glue ear. Is it the resolution of effusion in the middle ear, the restoration of pre-effusion hearing acuity, and the improvement of child behavior (a more "attentive," "responsive," and "alert" child)? If this is considered a sufficient justification for intervention (and for commitment of communal resources), the next question is, Have these effects been sufficiently demonstrated, and if so, in which children and under what conditions? If remediation of disease-current phenomena is considered the rationale for treatment, the answer to the question, What is it that we don't know and that matters, is, Not much, if anything. Several randomized controlled trials have established these disease-current benefits of surgical treatment of glue ear, although some controversy persists as to optimal treatment modality (ventilation tubes or adenoidectomy).

If, however, these treatment effects are considered not a sufficient reason for intervention, then the current information about glue ear is still true, but of limited relevance. If it is held that surgical intervention in the case of glue ear is warranted only if it helps to prevent developmental impairment, then there is still a lot that we don't know and that matters. Resolution of the effusion, restoration of hearing acuity, and reversal of behavioral changes are surrogate or intermediate end points at best, and they can never substitute for the real developmental end points. What, however, are realistic expectations with respect to the conclusiveness and timeliness of the results? What uncertainty tolerance is appropriate to the case at hand? Perhaps we would do better to accept the impossibility of conclusively establishing that persistent glue ear during childhood is developmentally compromising and that surgical treatment will prevent this. If the potential, or conceivable, effects of not treating the condition are far worse than those of treating it, then we might decide to continue current practice anyway. This benefit-of-the doubt approach is obviously the one followed by AHCPR.

Rarely, if at all, can such a discussion—of the treatment effects necessary to justify an intervention—be found in papers reporting the results of clinical trials. Such decisions have been made, of course, but usually in the study design and without further argumentation; they are implicit, for example, in the selected end points and the size of the study. For the most part, only after clinical trials are undertaken is it asked, Given this information, is the medical procedure worthwhile? A more principled discussion among stakeholders should, however, take place before starting a trial. Stakeholders include those persons involved in producing, using, and implementing the evaluation, those persons who profit in some way from the use of the evaluation, and those persons who may be negatively affected by the use of the evaluation.[41] When addressing the issues of the need for, and propriety of, a clinical trial, ideas concerning social justice and resource allocation in health care should not be ignored.[42] If it can be expected that there is difference of opinion on these issues within the professional community or between the professional community and other stakeholders (patient groups, policy makers), then the discussion should be brought to closure before embarking on the study. The issue is not trivial because of the vast amount of resources that are spent on evaluation studies, and the enrollment and randomization of patients in these studies. As in any other case, our resources (in terms of money, research capacity, and patients) are limited, and any trial has the cost of pursuing an opportunity. Therefore, a more accountable procedure for prioritizing evaluation studies is called for.

To be sure, concern has been expressed by assessors of medical technology about the limited impact of the results of their studies on medical practice. This has given an impetus to researchers to assess which criteria should be met by an assessment so as to increase the likelihood of a significant impact from its results. No doubt this is important, strategic research. But we should also ask, Which criteria should be met by an assessment so that we can legitimately expect compliance with its recommedations on the part of those who are involved? To me it seems that the value issues discussed here should be discussed more openly and more explicitly, and ideally resolved among stakeholders before a new study is started.

NOTES

1. David H. Banta, "Minimally Invasive Therapy in Europe: A Case of Conflicts between Policy Limitations, Physician Conservatism, and Patient Demands," in *Technology and Democracy: The Use and Impact of Technology Assessment in Europe,* Proceeding of the 3rd European Congress on Technology Assessment (Copenhagen, November 4–7, 1992), p. 103.

2. R. A. Bright et al., "The Prevalence of Tympanostomy Tubes in Children in the United States, 1988," *American Journal of Public Health* 83, no. 7 (1993): 1026–8.

3. J. H. Dempster, G. G. Browning, and S. G. Gatehouse, "A Randomized Study of the Surgical Management of Children with Persistent Otitis Media with Effusion Associated with a Hearing Impairment," *J. Laryngol Otol* (1993): 284–9; H. Stephenson and M. Haggard, "Rationale and Design of Surgical Trials for Otitis Media with Effusion," *Clin Otolaryngol* 17 (1992): 67–78.

4. S. E. Stool et al., *Managing Otitis Media with Effusion in Young Children: Quick Reference Guide for Clinicians,* AHCPR Publication No. 94-0623 (Rockville, Md.: AHCPR, 1994).

5. J. L. Northern and M. P. Downs, *Hearing in Children,* 4th edition (Baltimore; Williams and Wilkins, 1991).

6. E. Manders and J. Tyberghein, "The Effects of Ventilation Tube Placement on Hearing, Speech, Language, Cognition and Behaviour," *Acta Oto-Rhino-Laryngologica Belgica* 47, no. 1 (1993): 27–32.

7. *The Treatment of Persistent Glue Ear in Children,* Effective Health Care, no. 4 (Leeds, United Kingdom: University of Leeds, School of Public Health), 1992.

8. P. S. Roland et al., "Otitis Media: Incidence, Duration, and Hearing Status," *Arch Otolaryngol Head Neck Surg* 115 (1989): 1049–53.

9. J. O. Klein, D. W. Teele, and S. I. Pelton, "New Concepts in Otitis Media: Results of Investigations of the Greater Boston Otitis Media Study Group," *Advances in Pediatrics* 39 (1992): 127–56. The results of this study have been challenged by Paradise et al., "Secretory Otitis Media: What Effects on Children's Development?" in *The Child and the Environment: Present and Future Trends,* ed. R. Fior and G. Pestalozza (New York: Elsevier Science Publishers, 1993); Dempster, Browning, and Gatehouse, "A Randomized Study"; Stephenson and Haggard, "Rationale and Design" who argue that OME and the associated hearing impairment are not the cause of later-life

developmental impairments. Instead, these authors consider both OME and these impairments as the result of a common, multiple cause (genetic, perinatal, constitutional, socioeconomic, or environmental factors), predisposing children to early-life OME and later-life less than optimal development.

10. D. Chalmers et al., "Otitis Media with Effusion in Children: The Dunedin Study," *Clinics in Developmental Medicine* 108 (1989): 1–167.

11. J. E. Roberts et al., "Otitis Media in Early Childhood and Cognitive, Academic, and Classroom Performance of the School-Aged Child," *Pediatrics* 83, no. 4 (1989): 477–85; P. F. Wright et al., "Impact of Recurrent Otitis Media on Middle Ear Function, Hearing, and Language," *J of Pediatrics* 113, no. 3 (1988): 581–7; T. W. Hubbard et al., "Consequences of Unremitting Middle-Ear Disease in Early Life: Otologic, Audiologic, and Developmental Findings in Children with Cleft Palate," *NEJM* 312, no. 24 (1985): 1529–34; J. Lous, M. Fiellau-Nikolajsen, and A. L. Jeppesen, "Secretory Otitis Media and Language Development: A Six-Year Follow-up Study with Case-Control," *J of Pediatric Otorhinolaryngol,* 15: 185–203.

12. N. A. Black, "Fashion, Science, and Technical Change: The History of the Treatment of Glue Ear," *Clin Otolaryngol* 10 (1985): 31–41.

13. N. Black, "Surgery for Glue Ear—Modern Epidemic," *Lancet* (April 14, 1984): 835–7.

14. N. Black, "Glue Ear: The New Dyslexia?" *BMJ* 290 (1985): 1963–5.

15. N. Black, "Geographical Variations in Use of Surgery for Glue Ear," *J Royal Society of Medicine* 78 (1985): 641–8.

16. I. M. Smith, A. R. Maw, and M. Dilkes, "The Use of Ventilation Tubes in Secretory Otitis Media: A Review of Consultant Otolaryngologists," *Clin Otolaryngol* 16 (1991): 334–7.

17. I. M. Smith and A. R. Maw, "Secretory Otitis Media: A Review of Management by Consultant Otolaryngologists," *Clin Otolaryngol* 16 (1991): 266–70.

18. G. R. Close et al., "Variation in Selected Childhood Surgical Procedures: The Case of Tonsillectomy and Management of Middle Ear Disease," *J Paediatr Child Health* 29 (1993): 429–33.

19. P. Spilseth, "Appropriateness of Tympanostomy Tubes," *Family Practice Research Journal* 12, no. 1 (1992): 43–52.

20. L. C. Kleinman et al., "The Medical Appropriateness of Tympanostomy Tubes Proposed for Children Younger Than 16 Years in the United States," *JAMA* 271 (1994): 1250–5.

21. M. E. Johns, "The Medical Appropriateness of Tympanostomy Tubes Proposed for Children Younger than 16 Years in the United States," editorial comment, *Arch Otolaryngol Head Neck Surg* 120 (1994): 801–2.

22. N. A. Black et al., "A Randomized Controlled Trial for Surgery for Glue Ear," *BMJ* 300 (1990): 1551–6; E. M. Mandel et al., "Efficacy of Myringotomy with and without Tympanostomy Tubes for Chronic Otitis Media with Effusion," *Pediatr Infec Dis J* 11 (1992): 270–7; P. Bonding and M. Tos, "Grommets versus Paracentesis in Secretory Otitis Media, a Prospective Controlled Study," *Am J Otolaryngol* 6, no. 6 (1985): 455–60.

23. *Effective Health Care.*

24. T. Lildholdt, "Ventilation Tubes in Secretory Otitis Media: A Randomised, Controlled Study of the Course, the Complications, and the Sequelae of Ventilation Tubes," *Int J of Pediatric Otorhinolaryngol,* Suppl. 398 (1983): 185–203.

25. M. Tos and S. E. Stangerup, "Hearing Loss in Tympanosclerosis Caused by Grommets," *Arch Otolaryngol Head Neck Surg* 115 (1989): 931–5.

26. Manders and Tyberghein, "The Effects of Ventilation Tube Placement."

27. Northern and Downs, *Hearing in Children,* p. 65.

28. M. P. Haggard, G. G. Browning, and J. A. Birkin, "Effectiveness of Surgery for OME in 3.5–7 Year Olds on Multiple Developmental Outcomes—Piloting of a Large RCT Research Protocol," (Unpublished manuscript, 1993).

29. E. I. Cantekin et al., "Lack of Efficacy of a Decongestant-Antihistamine Combination for Otitis Media with Effusion ('Secretory' Otitis Media) in Children: Results of a Double-Blind, Randomized Trial," *NEJM* 308 (1983): 297–301.

30. E. M. Mandel et al., "Efficacy of Amoxicillin with and without Decongestant-Antihistamine for Otitis Media with Effusion in Children," *NEJM* 316 (1987): 432–7.

31. L. Widemar et al., "The Effect of Adenoidectomy on Secretory Otitis Media: A 2-Year Controlled Prospective Study," *Clin Otolaryngol* 10 (1985): 345–50; N. Roydhouse, "Adenoidectomy for Otitis Media with Mucoid Effusion," *Ann Otol Rhinol Laryngol* 89, Suppl. 68 (1980): 312–15; M. Fiellau-Nikolajsen, J. Falbe-Hansen, and P. Knudstrup, "Adenoidectomy for Middle Ear Disorders: A Randomized Controlled Trial," *Clin Otolaryngol* 5 (1980): 323–7.

32. C. H. Bulman, S. J. Brook, and M. G. Berry, "A Prospective Randomized Trial of Adenoidectomy vs. Grommet Insertion in the Treatment of Glue Ear," *Clin Otolaryngol* 9 (1984): 67–75.

33. Bolman, Brook, and Berry, "A Prospective Randomized Trial," p. 75.

34. G. A. Gates et al., "Effectiveness of Adenoidectomy and Tympanostomy Tubes in the Treatment of Chronic Otitis Media with Effusion," *NEJM* 317 (1987): 1444–51.

35. J. L. Paradise et al., "Secretory Otitis Media: What Effects on Children's Development?" in *The Child and the Environment: Present and Future Trends,* ed. R. Fior and G. Pestalozza (New York: Elsevier Science Publishers, 1993); Dempster, Browning, and Gatehouse, "A Randomized Study"; Stephenson and Haggard, "Rationale and Design."

36. Paradise et al., "Secretory Otitis Media."

37. R. J. Ruben, "Effectiveness and Efficacy of Early Detection of Hearing Impairment in Children," *Acta Otolaryngol* (Stockholm), Suppl. 482 (1991): 127–31.

38. R. J. Ruben, "An Inquiry into the Minimal Amount of Auditory Deprivation Which Results in a Cognitive Effect in Man," *Acta Otolaryngol* (Stockholm), Suppl. 414 (1984) 127–31.

39. R. H. Gaskins, *Burdens of Proof in Modern Discourse* (New Haven: Yale University Press, 1992).

40. Stool et al., "Managing Otitis Media."

41. E. G. Guba and Y. S. Lincoln, *Fourth Generation Evaluation* (Newbury Park, Calif.: Sage, 1989), pp. 40–1.

42. N. Daniels, *Just Health Care* (Cambridge: Cambridge University Press, 1985); J. Elster, *Local Justice: How Institutes Allocate Scarce Goods and Necessary Burdens* (Cambridge: Cambridge University Press, 1992); A. Heller, *Beyond Justice* (Oxford: Blackwell, 1987).

Donald J. Murphy

Guideline Glitches: Measurements, Money, and Malpractice

Expectations for outcomes data and resulting practice guidelines are high for many health care professionals. I, too, share enthusiasm for the critical analysis (i.e., outcomes research and guideline development) that has emerged over the last two decades, but I also have doubts about the promises of this movement.

From a clinician's perspective, I will focus on the practical obstacles to guidelines' reaching their potential. I choose guidelines because their recommendations for action are unequivocal. If guidelines are to enhance health care yet control costs, professionals and outcomes researchers must overcome most of these obstacles. Obstacles can be eliminated, but it won't be easy.

Many factors influence physicians' compliance with guidelines. These include their attitudes about utilization review,[1] government regulation,[2] physician profiling,[3] uncertainty,[4] private industry,[5] clinical autonomy,[6] sponsors of the guidelines,[7] necessity and appropriateness of care,[8] opinion leaders,[9] conflict in guidelines,[10] and the value of guidelines in general.[11] Patients' expectations[12] and the sociocultural milieu are other important factors.[13] No doubt many more factors exist that have not been studied.

This chapter focuses on three other factors that are frequently operative from a clinician's perspective. Investigators and clinicians are well aware of two of these factors, money and malpractice.[14] At some level, many physicians think about money and malpractice every day. The third factor, measurements, is not so obvious. A case study helps illustrate these three factors.

Case Study

Mrs. Hart is an eighty-five-year-old with diabetes, a history of breast cancer, and advanced coronary artery disease. She had an angioplasty in 1990. Her angina and shortness of breath were stable until September 1994, when these symptoms accelerated despite near maximal medical therapy. The attending physician referred Mrs. Hart to a cardiologist to see if she needed another angioplasty. The cardiologist interviewed and examined Mrs. Hart, did an

Guideline Glitches: Measurements, Money, and Malpractice 101

echocardiogram, and concluded that further medical intervention, including an angioplasty, was not indicated. He suggested a change of her medications.

Two months after the consultation, Mrs. Hart came to the emergency room having experienced eight hours of severe chest pain. She had a myocardial infarction (MI). The emergency room physicians decided not to use thrombolytics because eight hours had elapsed since the onset of her pain. The cardiologist said that Mrs. Hart had had a "small MI." After the first day in the hospital, she remained pain-free, and she had no more shortness of breath than usual. On the fourth hospital day the cardiology team ordered an echocardiogram. On the fifth day they ordered a thallium treadmill test. The attending physician decided to discharge Mrs. Hart without doing further tests.

Measurements

I, for one, am conflicted about measurements. On one hand, I support the move to make clinical decisions and guideline development more scientific, and this requires better measurements. On the other hand, we mislead ourselves when we confuse clinical decision making with science.[15] Sophisticated measurements may encourage automatic reflexes, not the artistry that good clinicians need.

I suggest we live with this ambivalence by addressing three fundamental questions about measurements. First, what should be measured? Second, how should it be measured? And third, how should the measurements be reported? Each of these questions requires much more attention than this essay can provide. My comments are limited to a caveat and a clinical example regarding each question.

What should be measured? Caveat number one: Let's not be seduced by technology (e.g., sophisticated statistics) when deciding what to measure. Alvan Feinstein's 1994 article, "Clinical Judgment Revisited: The Distraction of Quantitative Models,"[16] is an indictment of much of our recent clinical investigation on exactly this point. Feinstein claims that during the past couple of decades, clinical investigators have been seduced by "hard" data, randomized trials, Bayes theorem, quantitative decision analysis, psychometrics, and medical-claims administrative data.[17] No doubt, many analyses using these quantitative models have been very useful, but sophisticated statistics (e.g., logistic regression) have also enabled us to perform myriad analyses of little clinical significance. Feinstein stated, "Awed and baffled by the arcane vocabulary and statistics, clinical investigators may have neglected the appraisal of 'face validity'—a statistically unmeasurable attribute that refers to the measurement's clinical 'sensibility' or 'common sense' in doing its intended job."[18] Too often technology usurps the place of common sense or clinical sense.

Consider risk stratification. Statistical models allow us to identify the important prognostic factors for numerous clinical situations. Every month the cardiology literature has forty to fifty articles focusing on specific prognostic factors. With precise risk stratification, clinicians can tell their patients the likelihood that something bad will happen within a defined time period. If the risk seems too high and the risk can be modified (through medications, lifestyle changes, or a procedure), then the clinician and patient can use the information about prognostic factors to make an informed decision. This approach is fine as long as precision does not preempt common sense.

Mrs. Hart has advanced coronary artery disease. A cardiology guideline suggests that Mrs. Hart's clinicians should "risk stratify" her before she returns home after her MI. In other words, Mrs. Hart should have whatever tests are necessary to determine a precise prognosis. Specifically, Mrs. Hart and her clinicians should know the likelihood that she will have another MI in the next year. Information from an echocardiogram and a thallium treadmill test would make the prognosis more precise.

What's wrong with this approach? In this case, the precision gleaned from these tests does not matter. We are going to treat Mrs. Hart in the same fashion no matter what these tests reveal. What if we hadn't already maximized medical therapy for Mrs. Hart and were still considering an operation? Then wouldn't prognostic precision be desirable? Yes, of course it would be, but let's not forget common sense.

Several clinicians, including a cardiology team, took care of Mrs. Hart. No doubt the collective experience and knowledge of Mrs. Hart's doctors would have yielded a fairly accurate response to the question, What's the likelihood she will have a fatal MI in the next year? Assume a 20 percent chance. Assume, too, however, that the most precise answer in 1997 is actually 25 percent and that precision can only be obtained by doing an echocardiogram and thallium treadmill test. Does it matter? Mrs. Hart's decision would unlikely change if the answer was 25 percent (or 15 percent) instead of 20 percent. Common sense suggests that the difference between estimates from seasoned clinicians and those from prognostic models doesn't amount to much at the bedside. This singly underscores the conclusion that "the goal of risk stratification may be multibillion dollar care leading a potentially multibillion dollar horse in an unknown direction."[19] Unfortunately, a medical culture dominated by risk stratification and other quests for certainty will create guidelines that look very different from those focused on what matters for decision making among patients and doctors.

How should measurements be taken? Caveat number two: Beware of conveniently collected data that are supposed to measure complex decision making. The outcomes movement is full of survey instruments. Some are short and simple; others are long and complex. Completion of some surveys depends on research assistants collecting the data. Rarely do the patients' clinicians perform the surveys. This is a matter of convenience (clinicians don't have the time or interest to collect the data) or an attempt to minimize biases.

In the quest for objective data, scientists try to minimize all biases. Many think that an unbiased, outside observer (e.g., research assistant) can collect data more accurately than a biased physician who has known the patient for years; often many are misguided in this assumption.

Consider preferences regarding cardiopulmonary resuscitation (CPR). The literature is replete with studies suggesting that a fair percentage of seniors (10 to 30) would opt for CPR in the event of an advanced chronic disease such as Alzheimer's.[20] A study involving my patients at a geriatrics clinic indicates that only 5 percent of seniors would want CPR under the condition of chronic illness where the life expectancy was less than one year.[21] All of these studies—even the one involving my patients—overestimate the percentage of seniors opting for CPR. Why? Because physicians have approached this complex question as researchers, not as clinicians who have trusting relationships with patients. As a clinician, I believe the percentage of seniors who would want CPR in the setting of advanced dementia is less than 1 percent. I have talked with hundreds of seniors about CPR, and I know of only one who would want CPR regardless of her condition and prognosis. The experiences of my colleagues who routinely discuss advance directives similarly do not reflect what is reported in the medical literature.

I fully support the move to measure patient preferences.[22] A recent guideline that incorporates much counseling in the algorithm is a model that all guideline developers should consider.[23] Data about complex medical decisions and outcomes may not be as reliable when they are obtained outside a trusting relationship.

How do we report the measurements? Caveat number three: We should be more honest in reporting measurements to individuals. Researchers, the media, and practicing clinicians all tend to portray medical advances in a positive light. For example, I could tell one of my patients, "Yearly mammograms will decrease your risk of fatal breast cancer by 33 percent." Or I could say, "Seven thousand people like you would need to have yearly mammograms in order to prevent one premature cancer death." Both statements are fairly accurate.[24] Which statement is more likely to encourage my patient to comply with my recommendation of yearly mammograms?

When we report results using relative risk reductions, the value of what we recommend (e.g., lowering blood pressure, lowering cholesterol, taking estrogen, etc.) looks good. When we report absolute risk reductions, however, the value looks marginal.[25] Imagine, for example, a new medicine that lowers cholesterol. We'll call it CleanArteries. A study involves 100 subjects taking CleanArteries and 100 matched subjects taking placebo. After five years, four of the placebo subjects have had heart attacks, but only two of the CleanArteries subjects have had heart attacks. The professional journals and the public media will likely report this breakthrough as follows: "CleanArteries Reduces Your Risk of Heart Attack by 50 Percent." They are reporting the relative risk reduction (two is 50 percent of four) because a headline that reads, "CleanArteries May Reduce Risk of Heart Attack by 2 Percent" won't go very far in our culture. This, however, is the absolute risk reduction. Similarly, some seniors will opt for cancer screening when the detection rate is very low, and they will opt for prophylaxis when the absolute risk reduction is very low.[26] Many seniors, however, would not opt for these measures if they understood the true value for them.[27]

A medical resident working in our clinic had suggested that Mrs. Hart start a cholesterol-lowering agent four months before her heart attack. He was following a guideline he had read the week before. He told Mrs. Hart that the medicine could reduce her risk of a heart attack by 10–20 percent. If we can extrapolate data from younger males[28] to older females, then the medical resident was correct. The medical resident was focusing on Mrs. Hart's relative risk reduction. Her absolute risk reduction was closer to 1–2 percent.[29] After the resident shared this information with her—and told her about the cost of various medications—Mrs Hart decided that the cholesterol-lowering agent wasn't worth it for her. She didn't want to follow the guideline. When patients and clinicians consider absolute risk reduction (and other ways of looking at measurements, such as the number needed to treat to prevent one bad outcome),[30] they may disagree with the experts who establish guidelines.

The best guidelines are those that encourage clinicians to blend art and science.[31] Guidelines that try to be scientific by giving too much weight to outcomes measurements will be of little use to doctors and patients who strive to know and respect each other.

Money

Money matters. Financial incentives influence clinicians' behavior.[32] Any seasoned clinician who looks honestly at the profession knows that the role of financial incentives is probably greater than the medical literature suggests.

Guidelines that account responsibly for the influence of money (or time) will be more useful than those that ignore these influences.

To understand the influence of money in medicine, we must disabuse ourselves of a fantasy to which most of us cling. We want to believe that doctors care a great deal about our problems and care very little about other things. The fantasy is that the patient's welfare is *the* primary concern for the doctor. The reality, however, is that the patient's welfare is *a* primary concern for the doctor. Occasionally, doctors are filled with empathy and focus intently on the patient's problem, allowing no distractions to interfere with the ideal patient-physician encounter. More often than not, doctors have several things on their minds. What will the patients in the waiting room think if I take an extra fifteen minutes with Mrs. Hart? Why didn't my wife have a better understanding of what I said last night? Will I have time for the meeting this evening? I hope my son's soccer team wins this afternoon. The concerns that could potentially interrupt the ideal nexus are endless.

Successful clinicians are not necessarily the ones who are most empathic, most knowledgeable, most charismatic, or whatever other quality we fantasize about doctors. A successful clinician is one that can balance numerous concerns while acting as if Mrs. Hart's sore back is *the* most important matter. Successful clinicians embrace conflicts of interests (e.g., clinician's free time versus extra time for the patient) and deal with them; they do not try to eradicate them by holding onto the fantasy that the patient's welfare is all that matters.

Money represents the conflict of interest clinicians must live with every day. Not all of the conflicts have financial implications, but most do. Time costs money. Diagnostic tests cost money. Detailed notes cost money. Responsible guidelines should account for the reality of financial incentives and the inevitable conflicts of interest that clinicians deal with routinely. Let's return to Mrs. Hart's hospitalization and consider two decision points. The first is the decision about thrombolytic therapy when she presented to the emergency room with an MI. How might money matter in this decision? In an effort to decrease the hospital's pharmacy costs, the Pharmacy and Therapeutics Committee at the hospital may have encouraged the use of streptokinase as the thrombolytic of choice. Streptokinase is much less expensive than t-PA. On the other hand, a cardiologist who is a stockholder in the company that makes t-PA may have convinced himself, his colleagues, and the Pharmacy and Therapeutics Committee that t-PA is indeed superior to streptokinase and that it should be the thrombolytic of choice.

The second decision involved Mrs. Hart's evaluation after she had been in the hospital for three days. As noted above, she had an echocardiogram and an exercise treadmill test, but the additional information gained about her from these tests was marginal. In a fee-for-service world, the cardiologist profits financially from these tests. In a capitated system, the cardiologist and I, the primary care physician, may lose financially from the same tests. Guidelines regarding thrombolytics or tests for risk stratification may look very different coming from a capitated system or from a fee-for-service system. We can accept these different guidelines if we are honest and recognize that money—not just quality care—is a key factor in the guideline development. Indeed, if guidelines from indemnity insurance plans and from capitated plans are the same, then someone has ignored the influence of money. I am referring not only to the money that the medical industry pockets but also to the money that the insurance subscribers are trying to save.

Malpractice

Malpractice is the real "M" word. I believe the threat of malpractice may influence most clinicians' behavior as much as any factor except the welfare of the patient. Informal surveys of medical audiences suggest that clinicians spend 20 to 40 percent of their time (writing detailed notes, ordering extra tests or consultations, etc.) trying to avoid malpractice,[33] and guidelines may ultimately affect this liability of clinicians.[34]

The medical literature can only hint at the impact of malpractice on clinicians' behavior. Let's return to Mrs. Hart. One month after I discharged her, I still felt uncomfortable that I had rescinded the orders of my colleague the cardiologist. I asked to talk with him. We were both grateful that we could be honest about our concerns. I soon learned that measurements and money had little to do with his recommendation that Mrs. Hart get an echocardiogram and thallium treadmill test. These tests were simply the standard of care for someone who has just had an MI; if a cardiologist doesn't follow this standard, he or she may be liable for an adverse health outcome. Did the cardiologist really need to follow this standard? No, not in this case, but it is the perception of risk that influences behavior.

Another example illustrates this point. In Denver, we are developing guidelines regarding the use of futile and inappropriate intensive care.[35] I am confident that the professional and lay communities will reach consensus on a number of guidelines.[36] For example, the community will agree that CPR is not indicated for certain patients[37] or that intensive care is not indicated for patients in a persistent vegetative state.[38] But I doubt these guidelines will be used at all if professionals believe that following the guidelines increases their risk of malpractice. Numerous conversations with clinicians in Denver hospitals indicate that tort reform is essential for these guidelines to work.

In the next three years, GUIDe (Guidelines for Use of Intensive Care in Denver) will be spending as much effort on professional mediation and developing nonjudicial routes of conflict resolution as it will on the guidelines themselves.

Guidelines for Guideline Development

On the basis of what I have said here, I offer the following guidelines for developing guidelines:

1. Consider measurements from the patients' perspectives.
2. Consider incentives as important as rules.[39]
3. Consider the perception of legal liability.
4. Be modest; guidelines are just guidelines.[40]

NOTES

1. S. D. Goold et al., "Measuring Physician Attitudes toward Cost, Uncertainty, Malpractice, and Utilization Review," *J Gen Intern Med* 9 (1994): 544–9.

2. C. D. Naylor and A. A. Hollenberg, "Practice Guidelines and Professional Autonomy in a Universal Health Insurance System: The Case of Tissue Plasminogen Activator in Ontario," *Soc Sci Med* 31 (1990): 1327–36 (abstract).

3. E. J. Topol and R. M. Califf, "Scorecard Cardiovascular Medicine: Its Impact and Future Directions," *Ann Intern Med* 120 (1994): 65–70; H. G. Welch, M. E. Miller, and W. P. Welch, "Physician Profiling: An Analysis of Inpatient Practice Patterns in Florida and Oregon," *NEJM* 330 (1994): 607–12.

4. S. D. Goold et al., "Measuring Physician Attitudes towards Cost," pp. 544–9; J. P. Kassirer, "Our Stubborn Quest for Diagnostic Certainty: A Cause of Excessive Testing," *NEJM* 320 (1989): 1489–91; E. B. Beresford, "Uncertainty and the Shaping of Medical Decision," *Hastings Center Report* 21, no. 4 (1991): 6–11.

5. L. T. Cowley et al., "Magnetic Resonance Imaging Marketing and Investment: Tensions between the Forces of Business and the Practice of Medicine," *Chest* 105 (1994): 920–8.

6. S. R. Tunis et al., "Internists' Attitudes about Clinical Practice Guidelines," *Ann Intern Med* 120 (1994): 956–63.

7. M. N. Hill and C. S. Weisman, "Physicians' Perceptions of Consensus Reports," *Int J Tech Assess Health Care* 7 (1991): 30–41.

8. J. P. Kahan et al., "Measuring the Necessity of Medical Procedures," *Med Care* 32 (1994): 357–65; A. G. Ellrodt, M. Reidlinger, and S. Weingarten, "Measuring and Improving Physician Compliance with Clinical Practice Guidelines: A Controlled Interventional Trial," *Ann Intern Med* 122 (1995): 277–82.

9. J. Lomas et al., "Opinion Leaders vs Audit and Feedback to Implement Practice Guidelines: Delivery after Previous Cesarean Section," *JAMA* 265 (1991): 2202–7.

10. J. A. Charnow, "Can Guidelines Reflect the Realities of Daily Practice?" *American College of Physicians Observer* 10 (1990): 1–7.

11. A. G. Ellrodt, M. Reidlinger, and S. Weingarten, "Measuring and Improving Physician Compliance"; J. M. Grimshaw and I. T. Russell, "Effect of Clinical Guidelines on Medical Practice: A Systematic Review of Rigorous Evaluations," *Lancet* 342 (1993): 1317–22.

12. J. A. Charnow, "Can Guidelines Reflect the Realities?"

13. J. M. Eisenberg, "Sociologic Influences on Decisionmaking by Clinicians," *Ann Intern Med* 90 (1979): 957–64.

14. P. Boyle and D. Callahan, "Technology Assessment: The Missing Human Dimension," *Hastings Center Report* 22 (1992): 38–9; L. Goldman, "Changing Physicians' Behavior: The Pot and the Kettle," *NEJM* 322 (1990): 1524–5; P. J. Greco and J. M. Eisenberg, "Changing Physicians' Practices," *NEJM* 329 (1993): 1271–4.

15. E. B. Beresford, "Uncertainty and the Shaping."

16. A. R. Feinstein, "Clinical Judgment Revisited: The Distraction of Quantitative Models," *Ann Intern Med* 120 (1994): 799–805.

17. A. R. Feinstein, "Clinical Judgment Revisited."

18. A. R. Feinstein, "Clinical Judgment Revisited."

19. B. M. Massie and D. T. Mangano, "Assessment of Perioperative Risk: Have We Put the Cart before the Horse?" *J Am Coll Cardiol* 21 (1993): 1353–6.

20. R. S. Schonwetter et al.; "Educating the Elderly: Cardiopulmonary Resuscitation Decisions before and after Intervention," *J Am Geriatr Soc* 39 (1991): 372–7; C. Michelson et al., "Eliciting Medical Care Preferences from Nursing Home Residents," *Gerontologist* 31 (1991): 358–63; R. F. Uhlmann, R. A. Pearlman, and K. C. Cain, "Understanding of Elderly Patients' Resuscitation Preferences by Physicians and Nurses," *West J Med* 150 (1989): 705–7; M. A. Everhart and R. A. Pearlman, "Stability of Patient Preferences Regarding Life-Sustaining Treatments," *Chest* 97 (1990): 159–64.

21. D. J. Murphy et al., "The Influence of the Probability of Survival on Patients' Preferences Regarding Cardiopulmonary Resuscitation," *NEJM* 330 (1994): 543–9.

22. A. R. Feinstein, "Clinical Judgment Revisited"; G. A. Diamond and T. A. Denton, "Alternative Perspectives on the Biased Foundations of Medical Technology Assessment," *Ann Intern Med* 118 (1993): 455–64; M. Gillick, "The High Costs of Dying: A Way Out," *Arch Intern Med* 154 (1994): 2134–7.

23. D. C. Hadorn, K. McCormick, and A. Diokno, "An Annotated Algorithm Approach to Clinical Guideline Development," *JAMA* 267 (1992): 3311–4.

24. D. J. Murphy, *Honest Medicine: Shattering the Myths about Aging and Health Care* (New York: Atlantic Monthly Press, 1995).

25. D. J. Murphy, *Honest Medicine*, 1995; A. S. Brett, "Treating Hypercholesterolemia: How Should Practicing Physicians Interpret the Published Data for Patients?" *NEJM* 321 (1989): 676–80; D. J. Malenka et al., "The Framing Effect of Relative

and Absolute Risk," *J Gen Intern Med* 8 (1993): 543–8; L. Forrow, W. C. Taylor, and R. M. Arnold, "Absolutely Relative: How Research Results Are Summarized Can Affect Treatment Decisions," *Am J Med* 92 (1992): 121–4; C. D. Naylor, E. Chen, and B. Strauss, "Measured Enthusiasm: Does the Method of Reporting Trial Results Alter the Perceptions of Therapeutic Effectiveness?" *Ann Intern Med* 117 (1992): 916–21; H. C. Bucher and M. Weinbacher, "Influence of Method or Reporting Study Results on Decision of Physicians to Prescribe Drugs to Lower Cholesterol Concentration," *BMJ* 309 (1994): 761–4.

26. D. J. Murphy et al., "Seniors' Preferences for Screening and Prophylaxis Based on Absolute Risk Reduction," *J Am Geriat Soc* (1994): Supplement p. 63.

27. D. J. Murphy et al., "Seniors' Preferences."

28. Lipid Research Clinics Program, "The Lipid Research Clinics Coronary Primary Prevention Trial Results: I. Reduction in Incidence of Coronary Heart Disease," *JAMA* 251 (1984): 351–64.

29. A. S. Brett, "Treating Hypercholesterolemia"; Lipid Research Clinics Program, "Reduction in Incidence of Coronary Heart Disease."

30. D. J. Murphy, G. J. Povar, and L. G. Pawlson, "Setting Limits in Clinical Medicine," *Arch Intern Med* 154 (1994): 505–12.

31. A. L. Hillman, "Managing the Physicians: Rules Versus Incentives," *Health Affairs* 10, no. 4 (Winter 1991): 138–46.

32. K. M. Langa and E. J. Sussman, "The Effect of Cost-Containment Policies on Rates of Coronary Revascularization in California," *NEJM* 329 (1993): 1784–9; B. J. Hillman et al., "Physicians' Utilization and Charges for Outpatient Diagnostic Imaging in a Medicare Population," *JAMA* 268 (1992): 2050–4; A. M. Epstein, C. B. Begg, and B. J. McNeil, "The Use of Ambulatory Testing in Prepaid and Fee-for-Service Group Practices: Relation to Perceived Profitability," *NEJM* 314 (1986): 1089–94; A. L. Hillman, M. V. Pauly, and J. J. Kerstein, "How Do Financial Incentives Affect Physicians' Clinical Decisions and the Financial Performance of Health Maintenance Organizations?" *NEJM* 321 (1989): 86–92; B. J. Hillman et al., "Frequency and Cost of Diagnostic Imaging in Office Practice—A Comparison of Self-Referring and Radiologist-Referring Physicians," *NEJM* 323 (1990): 1604–8; D. Hemenwaym et al., "Physicians' Responses to Financial Incentives: Evidence from a For-Profit Ambulatory Care Center," *NEJM* 322 (1990): 1059–63; J. Lomas et al., "Do Practice Guidelines Guide Practice? The Effect of a Consensus Statement on the Practice of Physicians," *NEJM* 321 (1989): 1306–11.

33. D. J. Murphy, *Honest Medicine.*

34. J. A. Charnow, "Can Guidelines Reflect the Realities of Daily Practice?"; E. B. Hirshfeld, "Practice Parameters and the Malpractice Liability of Physicians," *JAMA* 263 (1990): 1556–62; E. B. Hirshfeld, "Should Practice Parameters Be the Standard of Care in Malpractice Litigation?" *JAMA* 266, no. 20 (1991): 2886–91; D. Jutras, "Clinical Practice Guidelines as Legal Norms," *Can Med Assoc J* 148 (1993): 905–8; D. W. Garnick, A. M. Hendricks, and T. A. Brennan, "Can Practice Guidelines Reduce the Number of Costs of Malpractice Claims?" *JAMA* 266 (1991): 2856–60;

S. H. Woolf, "Practice Guidelines: A New Reality in Medicine: III. Impact on Patient Care," *Arch Intern Med* 153 (1993): 2646–55.

35. D. J. Murphy and E. Barbour, "Guide (Guidelines for the Use of Intensive Care in Denver): A Community Effort to Define Futile and Inappropriate Care," *New Horizons* 2 (1994): 326–31.

36. D. J. Murphy, "The Public and the Profession: Meeting at the Right Place," *J Law Med Ethics* 22 (1994): 161–2.

37. D. J. Murphy and T. E. Finucane, "New Do-Not-Resuscitate Policies: A First Step in Cost Control," *Arch Intern Med* 153 (1993): 1641–8.

38. D. J. Murphy and E. Barbour, "A Community Effort."

39. A. L. Hillman, "Managing the Physicians."

40. A. M. Epstein, "Changing Physician Behavior: Increasing Challenges for the 1990s," *Arch Intern Med* 151 (1993): 1641–8; L. B. McGuire, "A Long Run for a Short Jump: Understanding Clinical Guidelines," *Ann Intern Med* 113 (1990): 705–8; P. E. Dans, "Credibility, Cookbook Medicine, and Common Sense: Guidelines and the College," *Ann Intern Med* 120 (1994): 966–8; C. J. McDonald and J. M. Overhage, "Guidelines You Can Follow and Can Trust: An Ideal and an Example," *JAMA* 271 (1994): 872–3; W. W. Parmley, "Clinical Practice Guidelines: Does the Cookbook Have Enough Recipes?" *JAMA* 272 (1994): 1374–5.

Susan E. Bell

Technology Assessment, Outcomes Data, and Social Context: The Case of Hormone Therapy

Technology assessment (TA) is a way to understand, evaluate, and make decisions about medical interventions.[1] It includes the determination of safety, efficacy, and effectiveness, as well as "consideration of quality of life and patients' preferences, and especially the evaluation of costs and benefits."[2] Technology assessment, in other words, "offers the essential bridge between basic research and development and prudent practical application of medical technology."[3] In this essay, I provide a sociological perspective on the meaning of TA and its relationship to medical practice. My aim is threefold: to explore the assumptions about science that guide the development of TA, to consider how these assumptions make possible, shape, and limit TA, and, finally, to consider the implications of this analysis for understanding the link between TA and medical practice. These topics are explored by examining two texts: a TA of the use of hormone therapy to prevent disease and prolong life in asymptomatic postmenopausal women,[4] and clinical guidelines—a series of recommendations and specifications—for treating postmenopausal women with hormone therapy based on this TA.[5]

My analysis draws upon recent historical and sociological scholarship that demonstrates the uncertainty of medical research and medical practice.[6] In some respects menopause is well understood, yet the study of menopause demonstrates how there are always elements of uncertainty in medical practice. For example, clinicians have prescribed hormone therapy in one form or another to women for almost sixty years, yet they still do not entirely understand the meaning of menopause or the role of estrogen in the development of menopausal symptoms.[7] At present, there is controversy in medicine over whether hormone therapy "should be used to treat menopausal symptoms for a short period of time, thereby reducing any risks associated with long-term treatment, or whether it should also be used to prevent future disease, thereby requiring longer treatment that could increase the risk of cancer."[8]

I also draw upon scholarship that demonstrates the complexity of the development and diffusion of medical technology, a process that is evolving over time, marked by uncertainty, and shaped by values and structures at the broadest levels of society as well as those in local environments.[9] Hormone therapy in menopause exemplifies this process. It has undergone constant modification, beginning with the use of natural and then synthetic estrogens for short-term treatment[10] and evolving into the use of combinations of estrogen and progestin for long-term treatment after menopause to prevent bone loss and cardiovascular disease and to protect against osteoporosis.[11] As this literature points out, it is difficult to assess medical technology that is constantly evolving. To complicate matters further, the methodologies used to assess medical technologies are themselves constantly changing.

Finally, I draw upon recent historical, philosophical, and sociological scholarship that has demonstrated the contingency of modern scientific knowledge.[12] According to this critique, "there is no way to think about the construction of scientific knowledge apart from the social processes in and through which that activity takes place."[13] In science, as in all scholarly work, knowledge is "endowed with the viewpoint of the author/subject, who in turn is situated within her/his personal *experience*, which is the temporal intersection of historical, institutional, national, and international actions and events both local and global."[14] The work that scientists do is shaped not only by "nature" but by beliefs, interests, and cultural norms.

Scientific knowledge does not and cannot simply mirror nature.[15] Data never "speak for themselves" but always "presume interpretation."[16] Scientific outcomes are negotiated, and to be able to participate in negotiation with one another, scientists must share a common language. The resolution of negotiation in science and the emergence of one theory over another do not necessarily indicate that the "winner" is a better representation of reality but, rather, that advocates for one representation have been more successful than advocates for another at advancing their claims.[17] Although "consensus is commonly achieved . . . it is rarely compelled by the forces of logic and evidence alone."[18] In turn, negotiability arises from the "underdetermination of theoretical interpretations by the evidence."[19] The philosophical thesis of underdetermination claims that "any theory can be maintained in the face of any evidence, provided that we make sufficiently radical adjustments elsewhere in our beliefs."[20] On every level, choices must be made about which questions to ask, which methods to use, and what counts as an acceptable answer.[21] These choices "are social *even as* they are cognitive and technical."[22]

Meta-analysis, a TA that pools estimates from clinical studies to determine summary relative risks, exemplifies the ways in which scientific knowledge is contingent. Current social-science scholarship suggests that using this methodology involves a series of choices that are social as well as technical, made by individuals who are members of particular communities. These individuals negotiate with one another about what constitutes proof, evidence, explanation, and success in the process of assessing different medical technologies.[23]

In sum, hormone therapy and its assessment provide an example of uncertainty and contingency in the development, use, and assessment of medical technologies, as well as the relationship among TA, clinical guidelines, and medical practice.

History of Hormone Therapy in Menopause

Since 1937, medical scientists have understood that estrogen can relieve discomforts associated with menopause (cessation of menstruation). Just which discomforts it relieves has been a continuing matter of dispute,[24] but today medical scientists generally agree that it provides short-term benefits in relieving hot flashes, insomnia resulting from vasomotor changes, and atrophic urogenital changes.[25] More controversial is the long-term use of estrogen or a combination of estrogen and progestin in asymptomatic women to prevent osteoporosis and cardiovascular disease.[26]

In 1941, the synthetic estrogen diethylstilbestrol (DES) was approved by the Food and Drug Administration (FDA) for relieving discomforts of menopause and several other conditions. A year later the FDA approved Premarin, an estrogen derived from the urine of pregnant horses, to treat menopausal symptoms. Simultaneously, menopause was defined as an estrogen deficiency disease.[27] This designation marked the beginning of the medicalization of menopause, defining it as a problem to be treated medically.[28] By the 1960s, with encouragement from the distribution of the best-selling book *Feminine Forever*,[29] estrogens were widely prescribed to women during and after menopause, not only for specific discomforts but to preserve youth, elevate their moods, and enhance their sexuality.[30] In 1975, estrogen was the fifth most frequently prescribed drug in the United States; in the same year a survey in Washington State found that 51 percent of all postmenopausal women had used estrogens for at least three months, with a median duration of over ten years.[31] After 1975, estrogen usage briefly declined following publication of two reports linking estrogens with endometrial cancer.

In 1979, the use of menopausal estrogens began to increase again. In 1982, retail pharmacies dispensed sixteen million prescriptions for menopausal estrogens (oral, transdermal, injectable, vaginal, and oral androgen-estrogen combinations) and in 1992, thirty-nine million. Recently, Wyeth-Ayerst

114   Part II: Outcomes Data

Laboratories estimated "that about seven million women, or one-quarter of the 26.2 million women between 45–64 years old, are taking menopausal hormones."[32] In 1992, Wyeth-Ayerst's "Premarin became the most frequently dispensed brand-name pharmaceutical in the United States."[33] Sales of Premarin in 1993 totaled $644.2 million.[34] Because estrogen increases the risk of endometrial cancer, the American College of Obstetricians and Gynecologists recommends combining progestin with estrogen, either cyclically or continuously.[35] Histological, clinical, and epidemiological data "suggest that the addition of progestin to estrogen prevents the increase in endometrial cancer risk associated with estrogen therapy."[36] The FDA, however, has never approved the use of progestin for menopausal or postmenopausal use because its long-term effects and the lowest effective dosage for menopausal and postmenopausal women remain unknown.[37] Even so, once drugs are approved for any purpose by the FDA, physicians may prescribe these drugs beyond their approved uses "based on sound scientific evidence or medical opinion."[38] Between 1982 and 1992, prescriptions for oral progesterones (oral medroxyprogesterone) increased 4.9-fold, from 2.3 million in 1982 to 11.3 million in 1992.[39] This rate of growth is even faster than the rate of growth in prescriptions for menopausal estrogens, probably because of the protection from endometrial cancer that they may provide.

Today, unopposed estrogens are used much more commonly than combinations of estrogen and progestin, and they are used more widely by women who have had hysterectomies than by women who have intact uteri. According to the Office of Technology Assessment (OTA), in 1992 there were sixteen estrogen products marketed to treat symptoms of menopause, manufactured by twelve different pharmaceutical companies. By 1995, the FDA had approved four menopausal estrogens for long-term prevention of osteoporosis.[40] There were six progestin products marketed singly or in combination with estrogens by five manufacturers to treat symptoms of menopause in 1992.[41]

If physicians follow the clinical guidelines published by the American College of Physicians in 1992 and prescribe hormone therapy to asymptomatic postmenopausal women, the number of women taking hormones could be expected to rise even if the size of the population of older women were to remain constant. The number of women in the U.S. between the ages of forty-five and sixty-four is increasing, however, and so is the number of women aged sixty-five and older. Whereas at the turn of the century there were fewer than five million women fifty years old or older, by 1970 there were twenty-seven million (13 percent of the population), and by 1992 thirty-six million (14 percent of the population).[42] With a life expectancy of about eighty, women can expect to live thirty years after menopause (fifty is the average age at which menopause occurs in the United States).[43]

The Social and Cultural Context of Hormone Therapy

In the United States, women have historically lived longer than men but have been "sicker" than men, both objectively and subjectively.[44] With increasing numbers of women living longer lives and an expanding proportion of older women in the population, scholars have identified concomitant transformations in health research, policy, technology, and organization. Part of this transformation is reflected in the expanding market for "products and services that promise to delay or eliminate the supposed physiological effects of aging,"[45] including hormone therapy.

The increasing prescription of hormone therapy to women before and after menopause has been more than a response to the increasing numbers of menopausal and postmenopausal women. Rather, the development and diffusion of hormone therapy has been shaped by the larger social and cultural context of U.S. society. The first context that has influenced the development and diffusion of hormone therapy is the medicalization of aging in general and of menopause in particular. According to Carroll Estes and Elizabeth Binney,[46] the medicalization (or what they call "biomedicalization") of aging consists of "two closely related aspects: (1) the social construction of aging as a medical problem," that is, thinking of aging in terms of medical categories, and (2) the behaviors and policies in science, medical education, the government, and the lay public generally, based upon the conception of aging as a medical problem. That is, the medical worldview "takes precedence over, and in many cases defines, the basic biological, social, and behavioral processes and problems of aging" and "has influenced everything else—other research, policymaking, and the way we think about aging and even science."[47]

For women, the medicalization of aging is exemplified by the medicalization of menopause: defining it as a deficiency disease to be treated by physicians and transforming practice concomitantly.[48] In turn, the medicalization of menopause was made possible in part by reductionist assumptions about the role of hormones in women's behavior, sexist cultural norms about the proper role of aging women, and the availability of natural and synthetic hormones.[49] The medicalization of menopause reflected and reinforced the theory of hormone therapy, first in symptomatic menopausal women for short periods of time, then in all menopausal women, and currently, in addition, for specific categories of asymptomatic postmenopausal women for extended periods of time.

A second context shaping the development and diffusion of hormone therapy, related to the first, is a modern approach to understanding health and disease, predicated on the tenets of Western science. These tenets include objectivity, value neutrality, and controlled experimentation. Even though research based upon the assumptions of modern science has successfully led to some knowledge about the transition from reproductive to nonreproductive life, this research is systematically limited. As with its study of aging more generally, the modern approach to understanding health and disease focuses attention on biological and psychological processes associated with menopause in individuals and attempts to isolate, understand the etiology of, and intervene in these processes. The consequence of this focus is that it limits consideration of larger social and environmental factors in the experiences of menopausal and postmenopausal women and reduces "a complex phenomenon, its solution, and the public policy agenda in terms of medical problems and issues."[50] This has led to studies of menopause that focus "on single organ systems rather than on a [woman's] total physical and mental well-being" and on "single factors," such as medical interventions with hormone therapy, "rather than on a consideration of a [woman's] total way of life."[51]

A third context that has shaped the development and diffusion of hormone therapy for menopausal and postmenopausal women is Western capitalism. According to Howard Waitzkin,[52] in order to survive, "capitalist industries must produce and sell new products. Expansion is an absolute necessity for capitalist enterprises. The economic surplus . . . must grow continually larger." Pharmaceutical companies, like other capitalist industries, must continually enlarge their surplus value (profit); one of the ways this occurs is through the constant expansion of markets. Pharmaceutical companies have promoted the use of hormone therapy in various ways, with a great deal of success.[53] For example, even though none of the progestins used in combined hormone therapy has been approved for the treatment of menopausal symptoms, pharmaceutical companies have promoted the use of progestins beyond their FDA-approved and/or scientifically proven effects in the interest of profits.[54]

These three contexts shape the pace and direction of medical technology development and diffusion in general and hormone therapy in particular. They have guided the questions asked, the tools used to ask these questions, the collection and interpretation of data, and the representation and use of results.[55]

Meta-analysis of Hormone Therapy in Asymptomatic Postmenopausal Women

Like the development and diffusion of hormone therapy during and after menopause, the assessment of hormone therapy is also shaped by the larger social and cultural context of U.S. society. That is, the type of assessment chosen, the questions addressed, the interpretation and use of results are all reflections of medicalization, the modern approach to understanding health and disease, and the political economy. This connection is visible in the meta-analysis of the risks and benefits of the long-term use of hormone therapy in asymptomatic postmenopausal women.

Meta-analysis is a method of TA that pools estimates from studies in order to determine summary relative risks of specific technologies. In addition, it often provides detailed accounts of the data and criteria for inclusion of data sources, and assumptions used in the analysis.[56] In this way, meta-analysis makes sense out of a sometimes confusing array of reports, revealing the shortcomings of individual reports and putting them into a form in which they can be compared. What current social-science scholarship suggests, however, is not only that uncertainty will always be present in medicine but also that tools such as meta-analysis can mask that uncertainty in the language of objectivity, distance, and statistical analysis.

In the meta-analysis of hormone therapy in asymptomatic postmenopausal women, Deborah Grady and her associates critically reviewed the English-language literature published since 1970.[57] They assessed end points linked with hormone therapy that are major contributors to morbidity and mortality. Thus, they considered the effects of estrogen therapy and combinations of estrogen and progestin on endometrial cancer, breast cancer, coronary heart disease, osteoporosis, and stroke. They found "evidence that estrogen therapy decreases risk for coronary heart disease and for hip fracture, but long-term estrogen therapy increases risk for endometrial cancer and may be associated with a small increase in risk for breast cancer."[58] Other effects of long-term hormone therapy in asymptomatic women were less clear-cut. "The increase in endometrial cancer risk can probably be avoided by adding a progestin to the estrogen regimen for women who have a uterus, but the effects of combination hormones on risk for other diseases has [sic] not been adequately studied."[59] These results are consistent with the findings of a case study of menopause and its management conducted by the Office of Technology Assessment.[60]

On the basis of the meta-analysis, the American College of Physicians developed clinical guidelines for treating postmenopausal women with preventive hormone therapy.[61] Deborah Grady, senior author of the meta-analysis, was also the senior author of the clinical guidelines, which contain five recommendations: (1) "All women, regardless of race, should consider preventive hormone therapy." (2) "Women who have had a hysterectomy are likely to benefit from estrogen therapy." (3) "Women who have coronary heart disease or who are at increased risk for coronary heart disease are likely to benefit from hormone therapy" (but women with an intact uterus should be given combined hormone therapy). (4) For women at increased risk for breast cancer "the risks of hormone therapy may outweigh its benefits." (5) "For other women, the best course of action is not clear."[62] It is too early to tell what the effect of the guidelines has been on the use of hormone therapy in asymptomatic postmenopausal women.

Sociologically what is most striking about this meta-analysis are the authors' cautions about the limitations of their study. First, they caution that "in the absence of definitive evidence, [they] used the 'best' estimate of the change in risk for various diseases associated with hormone therapy."[63] With this caution, they acknowledge the role of judgment and uncertainty in the construction of scientific knowledge.

Second, the authors of the meta-analysis warn that "many estrogens and progestins are available, and regimens for combining progestin with estrogen are evolving. Use of different types or regimens of hormone therapy could affect our conclusions, as could new data on the effects of estrogen plus progestin regimens on risk for CHD, stroke, and breast cancer."[64] That is, the authors underscore the difficulties of assessing continuously evolving technologies.

Third, the authors write that "perhaps the greatest weakness of our assessment is that we did not evaluate the effect of therapy on quality of life, which may be the most important consideration for many women."[65] That is, they explicitly recognize a limitation of this meta-analysis.

The omission of quality of life as an aspect of studying the long-term use of hormone therapy is significant in at least three ways. First, there is evidence that women "afford greater weight to considerations of quality of life over quantity of life" when making decisions about hormone therapy.[66] That is, "women give high priority to the short-term impact of hormone therapy on their lives and do not make their decisions based on the risks of morbidity and mortality."[67] Second, although "hormone therapy is expected to reduce the risk of coronary heart disease and hip fracture and to extend life expectancy . . . the impact of these changes on quality of life is not clear."[68] Third, by excluding study of the impact of hormone therapy on quality of life, the meta-analysis is reflecting and repeating a pattern of exclusion in technology assessment more generally.[69]

The authors' caution about their omission of quality of life leads to the crux of the matter and can be translated into several types of questions: First, how can quality of life be put into the equation? Second, how can the quality-of-life experiences of individual women be measured and put into a "discourse" that will enable them to be evaluated in the same way as the effects of hormones on their bodies? Is putting their experiences into this "discourse" or "voice" possible? And third, is the discourse represented by technology assessment in general and meta-analysis in particular the best discourse for making judgments about clinical practice?

The meta-analysis embodies what has been called "the voice of medicine."[70] This voice seeks to understand and explain events within the framework of biomedicine, using the biomedical model.[71] According to the biomedical model, disease is a deviation from measurable biological functioning. Each disease has a specific etiology and a universal taxonomy. That is, diseases have identities separate from the particular bodies in which they develop, and disease processes "are basically indifferent to the value of their inhabitants." Thus, culture "is basically external to biology and disease."[72]

The biomedical model relies on modern science as the measure of truth. Accordingly, physicians strive to incorporate the scientific values of rationality, objectivity, and neutrality into their work. Even though these values "may be difficult to achieve in practice, nevertheless they retain their force as the basis for assessing the quality of clinical work."[73] For the voice of medicine, knowledge comes from "withdrawing from the noise and the crowds" of everyday life and from taking on a universal standpoint.[74] The physician as scientist disengages from "society, culture, emotion, and particular time and place."[75] The effect of the voice of medicine is to "strip away" the social context of health and illness as well as to ignore patients' self-understandings of their problems.[76]

A competing way of understanding and explaining disease and illness is the voice of the lifeworld.[77] The voice of the lifeworld maintains a connection between the body and the person. According to this voice, events become connected and meaningful depending on a person's "biographical situation and position in the social world."[78] The self is the center of the lifeworld. This voice contests the assumptions of the biomedical model. For example, although the cessation of menstruation is a universal biological experience, women's experience of their bodies during menopause is not universal; menopause is "a life-cycle transition to which powerful symbolic meanings, individual and social are attached."[79] Women's experiences of their bodies during menopause are not universal. In Japan, hot flashes are uncommon in most women (a recent survey found less than 20 percent of Japanese women ages forty-five to fifty-five had ever had hot flashes), and there is no Japanese word that refers uniquely to a hot flash. By contrast, in the United States, hot flashes are the sign most commonly associated with menopause (in 47 to 85 percent of women according to surveys).[80] These cultural differences suggest a relationship between the biology of menopause and the social meanings attached to aging, a connection that is sought by the voice of the lifeworld and severed by the voice of medicine.

Typically, the voice of medicine and the voice of the lifeworld are portrayed as being opposed: one embodied in the physician (or epidemiologist or biomedical scientist) and the other in the patient. Yet increasingly, scholars are demonstrating the extent to which the voices can be seen within each world.[81] A good example of this lies within the meta-analysis itself: the cautions by Grady and her coauthors might be read as acknowledgments of another way of seeing the world, of the difficulty of using both "voices" simultaneously, and perhaps (in the best of possible interpretations) of the necessity of using both. Another example can be found in the study of Japanese women, which makes the recommendation that "[t]ools for quantitative research must be culturally relevant; standard symptom lists in connection with menopause . . . are inadequate for cross-cultural studies."[82]

Technology Assessment Revisited

In the foregoing discussion, I have briefly sketched out the history of hormone therapy, the three contexts influencing the development and diffusion of hormone therapy as well as its assessment, and their connection with tensions contained and expressed within the recent meta-analysis of studies of the long-term use of hormone therapy in asymptomatic postmenopausal women. On the basis of that discussion, I would like to speculate about some of the ways that hormone therapy research, as well as assessments of that research, might be reformed to reflect more adequately the voices both of medicine and of the lifeworld.

First, the medicalization of menopause has directed attention to hormonal responses to the biological changes in women's bodies as a way of addressing the long-term health needs of aging women. Thus, a comparatively large number of studies have been conducted about the short- or long-term effects of hormone therapy on symptoms of menopause, osteoporosis, coronary heart disease, stroke, and endometrial and breast cancer. Comparatively few studies, however, have examined the effects of changes in diet, exercise, a woman's environment, and drugs other than estrogen or progestin on symptoms of menopause or on preventing disease and prolonging life in postmenopausal women.[83] Expanding the base of research could have the beneficial consequence not only of improving the science upon which clinical judgments are made regarding whether, when, and how to use hormone therapy in asymptomatic postmenopausal women, but also of resisting the medicalization of menopause from inside medicine.

Second, the tenets of modern science have fostered research methodologies that systematically exclude the voice of the lifeworld. The expansion of the research base to include study of health-related quality of life (QOL) would appear to be a mechanism for including that voice. Studies of QOL, however, typically exclude it. For example, in their review of the literature about health-related quality of life, sociologists Debra Lerner and Sol Levine[84] write that even the most inclusive models of QOL are too heavily influenced by "the still vibrant biomedical model" and thus they "decontextualize health-related QOL by treating bodily states and their consequences as problems intrinsic to individuals." Standard models of QOL have uncovered "very slippery problems which are associated with unraveling human values and ascribing an objective basis to them."[85] In other words, attempts to give voice to the concerns of the lifeworld in the voice of medicine are fraught with difficulty. The struggle to give them voice, and the possibility of determining the effects of hormone therapy on quality of life, however, may have the consequence of making the research more responsive to women's concerns and of contributing to a reform and transformation of Western science without rejecting it altogether.

Both of these speculations about transforming research refer to gaps in the body of research about hormone therapy and not about technology assessments about this research. But they have implications both for reforming technology assessment and for rethinking the connection between technology assessment and medical practice. First, both of them imply the need for even more reflexivity than is exemplified by the cautions made by Deborah Grady and her colleagues in their meta-analysis. Second, both imply the need for more acknowledgment of uncertainty and the use of judgment in all technology assessments. And third, they imply the need for finding ways to include the framework of the lifeworld in evaluating all medical technologies.

The translation from meta-analysis to clinical guidelines is one way to encourage the effective utilization of technology assessments. But the link between technology assessment and clinical practice is a complicated and tenuous one, as others have demonstrated in some detail.[86] In this essay, I have excluded study of this particular link in favor of exploring how the larger social, cultural, and economic contexts systematically influence technology assessments. In my view, understanding the social construction of technology assessments themselves can contribute to an understanding of how and why caregivers and their patients respond to the results of technology assessment results.

NOTES

1. Victor R. Fuchs and Allan M. Garber, "The New Technology Assessment," *NEJM* 323, no. 10 (1990): 673–7.

2. Fuchs and Garber, "The New Technology," p. 673.

3. Committee for Evaluating Medical Technologies in Clinical Use, Division of Health Sciences Policy, Division of Health Promotion and Disease Prevention,

Institute of Medicine, *Assessing Medical Technologies* (Washington, D.C.: National Academy Press, 1985), p. 70.

4. Deborah Grady et al., "Hormone Therapy to Prevent Disease and Prolong Life in Postmenopausal Women," *Annals of Internal Medicine* 117, no. 12 (1992): 1016–37.

5. American College of Physicians, "Guidelines for Counseling Postmenopausal Women about Preventive Hormone Therapy," *Annals of Internal Medicine* 117, no. 12 (1992): 1038–41.

6. Renée R. Anspach, *Deciding Who Lives* (Berkeley, Calif.: University of California Press, 1993); Susan E. Bell, "From Local to Global: Resolving Uncertainty about the Safety of DES in Menopause," *Research in the Sociology of Health Care* 11 (1994): 41–56; Susan E. Bell, "Translating Science to the People: Updating the New Our Bodies, Ourselves," *Women's Studies International Forum* 17, no. 1 (1994): 9–18; Elliot G. Mishler, *The Discourse of Medicine* (Norwood, N.J.: Ablex, 1984); Marianne A. Paget, *A Complex Sorrow: Reflections on Cancer and an Abbreviated Life* (Philadelphia, Penn.: Temple University Press, 1993); Paul Starr, *The Social Transformation of American Medicine* (New York: Basic Books, 1982).

7. U.S. Congress, Office of Technology Assessment, *The Menopause, Hormone Therapy, and Women's Health,* (Washington, D.C.: U.S. Government Printing Office, May 1992).

8. John H. Gibbons, "Foreword," in U. S. Congress, *The Menopause*, p. iii.

9. Susan E. Bell, "Technology in Medicine: Development, Diffusion, and Health Policy," in *Handbook of Medical Sociology, Fourth Edition,* ed. Howard E. Freeman and Sol Levine (Englewood Cliffs, N.J.: Prentice Hall, 1989), pp. 185–204; Howard Waitzkin, "A Marxian Interpretation of the Growth and Development of Coronary Care," in *The Sociology of Health and Illness: Critical Perspectives,* ed. Peter Conrad and Rochelle Kern (New York: St. Martin's Press, 1994), pp. 243–55.

10. S. Bell, "Changing Ideas: The Medicalization of Menopause," *Social Sciences and Medicine* 24, no. 6 (1987): 535–42; S. Bell, "Sociological Perspectives on the Medicalization of Menopause," *Annals of the New York Academy of Sciences* 592 (1990): 173–8.

11. U.S. Congress, *The Menopause;* American College of Obstetricians and Gynecologists, "Hormone Replacement Therapy," in *ACOG Technical Bulletin* no. 166 (Washington, D.C.: American College of Obstetricians and Gynecologists, April 1992); American College of Obstetricians and Gynecologists, "Osteoporosis," in *ACOG Technical Bulletin* no. 167 (Washington, D.C.: American College of Obstetricians and Gynecologists, May 1992).

12. Donna Haraway, "Situated Knowledges: The Science Question in Feminism and the Privilege of Partial Perspective," *Feminist Studies* 14 (1988): 575–99; Evelyn Fox Keller, *Reflections on Gender and Science* (New Haven, Conn.: Yale University Press, 1985); Bruno Latour and Steve Woolgar, *Laboratory Life: The Social Construction of Scientific Facts* (Beverly Hills, Calif.: Sage Publications, 1979).

13. E. Richards and J. Schuster, "The Feminine Method as Myth and Accounting

Resource: A Challenge to Gender Studies and Social Studies of Science," *Social Studies of Science* 19 No. 4 (1989): 697–720.

14. Joan H. Fujimura, "On Methods, Ontologies, and Representation in the Sociology of Science: Where Do We Stand?" in *Social Organization and Social Process,* ed. D. R. Maines (New York: Aldine DeGruyter, 1991), p. 217.

15. There is a voluminous literature about this point, beginning with Thomas S. Kuhn, *The Structure of Scientific Revolutions* (Chicago: University of Chicago, 1962). As Evelyn Fox Keller reminds us, however, even though this point has "come to seem obvious to many observers of science, they continue to seem largely absurd to the men and women actually engaged in the production of science." Evelyn Fox Keller, *Secrets of Life Secrets of Death: Essays on Language, Gender, and Science* (New York: Routledge, 1992), p. 26.

16. Keller, *Secrets of Life,* p. 27.

17. Keller, *Reflections;* Latour and Woolgar, *Laboratory Life.*

18. Keller, *Secrets of Life,* p. 26.

19. Karin D. Knorr-Cetina and Michael Mulkay, "Introduction: Emerging Principles in Social Studies of Science," in *Science Observed,* ed. Karin D. Knorr-Cetina and Michael Mulkay (Beverly Hills: Sage Publications, 1983), p. 12.

20. Knorr-Cetina and Mulkay, "Introduction," p. 3.

21. Keller, *Secrets of Life,* p. 31.

22. Keller, *Secrets of Life,* p. 26.

23. Keller, *Secrets of Life.*

24. Bell, "Changing Ideas"; U.S. Congress, *The Menopause.*

25. U.S. Congress, *The Menopause.*

26. Grady et al., "Hormone Therapy"; Lynn Rosenberg, "Hormone Replacement Therapy: The Need for Reconsideration," *American Journal of Public Health* 83, no. 12 (1993): 1670–3.

27. Bell, "Changing Ideas."

28. Bell, "Sociological Perspectives."

29. Robert N. Wilson, *Feminine Forever* (New York: Pocket Books, 1966).

30. U.S. Congress, *The Menopause.*

31. Frances B. McCrea, "The Politics of Menopause: The 'Discovery' of a Deficiency Disease," *Social Problems* 31 (1983): 111–13.

32. Diane K. Wysowski, Linda Golden, and Laurie Burke, "Use of Menopausal Estrogens and Medroxyprogesterone in the United States, 1982–1992," *Obstetrics & Gynecology* 85, no. 1 (1995): 9.

33. Wysowski, Golden, and Burke, "Use of Menopausal Estrogens," p. 7.

34. *Marketletter,* October 24, 1994.

35. American College of Obstetricians and Gynecologists, "Hormone Replacement."; American College of Obstetricians and Gynecologists, "Osteoporosis."

36. Grady et al., "Hormone Therapy," p. 1018.

37. Wysowski, Golden, and Burke, "Use of Menopausal Estrogens," p. 6.

38. U.S. Congress, *The Menopause,* p. 64.

39. Wysowski, Golden, and Burke, "Use of Menopausal Estrogens," p. 8.
40. Wysowski, Golden, and Burke, "Use of Menopausal Estrogens," p. 6.
41. U.S. Congress, *The Menopause*, chapter 4.
42. U.S. Bureau of the Census, *Statistical Abstract of the United States: 1994* [114th edition] (Washington, D.C.: Government Printing Office, 1994).
43. U.S. Congress, *The Menopause*, p. 3.
44. National Center for Health Statistics, *Health, United States 1992* (Hyattsville, Md.: Public Health Service, 1993).
45. Carrol L. Estes and Elizabeth A. Binney, "The Biomedicalization of Aging: Dangers and Dilemmas," *Gerontologist* 29, no. 5 (1989): 594.
46. Estes and Binney, "The Biomedicalization of Aging," p. 587.
47. Estes and Binney, "The Biomedicalization of Aging," p. 588.
48. Bell, "Changing Ideas"; McCrea, "The Politics of Menopause."
49. Bell, "Changing Ideas."
50. Estes and Binney, "The Biomedicalization of Aging," p. 589.
51. Rosenberg, "Hormone Replacement Therapy," p. 1671.
52. Waitzkin, "A Marxian Interpretation," p. 264.
53. U.S. Congress, *The Menopause*.
54. Waitzkin, "A Marxian Interpretation"; U.S. Congress, *The Menopause*.
55. Susan E. Bell, "A New Model of Medical Technology Development: A Case Study of DES," *Research in the Sociology of Health Care* 4 (1986): 1–32; Bell, "Changing Ideas"; Bell, "From Local to Global."
56. Fuchs and Garber, "The New Technology"; Grady et al., "Hormone Therapy."
57. Grady et al., "Hormone Therapy," p. 1016.
58. Grady et al., "Hormone Therapy," p. 1016.
59. Grady et al., "Hormone Therapy," p. 1016.
60. U.S. Congress, *The Menopause*.
61. American College of Physicians, "Guidelines."
62. American College of Physicians, "Guidelines," p. 1038.
63. Grady et al., "Hormone Therapy," p. 1030.
64. Grady et al., "Hormone Therapy," p. 1030.
65. Grady et al., "Hormone Therapy," pp. 1029–30.
66. U.S. Congress, *The Menopause*, p. 105.
67. U.S. Congress, *The Menopause*, p. 105.
68. Grady et al., "Hormone Therapy," p. 1030.
69. Debra J. Lerner and Sol Levine, "Health-Related Quality of Life: Origins, Gaps, and Directions," *Advances in Medical Sociology* 5 (1994): 43–65.
70. Mishler, *The Discourse of Medicine*.
71. Elliot G. Mishler, "Viewpoint," in *Social Contexts of Health, Illness, and Patient Care*, ed. E. G. Mishler et al. (Cambridge: Cambridge University Press, 1981), pp. 1–23.
72. Deborah R. Gordon, "Tenacious Assumptions in Western Medicine," in *Biomedicine Examined*, ed. Margaret Lock and Deborah Gordon (Boston: Kluwer Academic Press, 1988), pp. 19–56 at 28.

73. Mishler, "Viewpoint," pp. 15–16.
74. Gordon, "Tenacious Assumptions," p. 32.
75. Gordon, "Tenacious Assumptions," p. 33.
76. Mishler, *The Discourse of Medicine,* p. 120.
77. Mishler, *The Discourse of Medicine.*
78. Mishler, *The Discourse of Medicine,* p. 104.
79. Margaret Lock, "Contested Meanings of the Menopause," *Lancet* 337 (1991): 1270–2 at 1272.
80. F. Kronenberg, "Hot Flashes: Epidemiology and Physiology," *Annals of the New York Academy of Sciences* 592 (1990): 52–86; M. Flint, F. Kronenberg, and W. Utian eds., *Multidisciplinary Perspectives on Menopause* (New York: New York Academy of Sciences, 1990), 52–86.
81. Susan E. Bell and Roberta J. Apfel, "Looking at Bodies," *Qualitative Sociology* 18, no. 1 (1995): 3–19.
82. Lock, "Contested Meanings of the Menopause," p. 1272.
83. U.S. Congress, *The Menopause*; Rosenberg, "Hormone Replacement Therapy."
84. Lerner and Levine, "Health-Related Quality of Life," p. 52.
85. Lerner and Levine, "Health-Related Quality of Life," p. 62.
86. See, for example, Committee for Evaluating Medical Technologies in Clinical Use, *Assessing Medical Technologies,* chapter 4.

Susan E. Kelly and Barbara A. Koenig

"Rescue" Technologies following High-Dose Chemotherapy for Breast Cancer: How Social Context Shapes the Assessment of Innovative, Aggressive, and Lifesaving Medical Technologies

Introduction

In 1995, two women at Dana-Farber Cancer Institute were given accidental overdoses of chemotherapy as they underwent experimental high-dose treatment for metastatic breast cancer. One woman died, the other was seriously injured.[1] The goal of high-dose chemotherapy is to kill the maximum number of cancer cells; the drugs used are so potent they destroy not only the malignant cells but the patient's own blood-producing system as well. Even at conventional levels, the drugs given are highly toxic. Experimental high-dose chemotherapy requires doses so large the patient must subsequently be "rescued" by infusion of new bone marrow or blood-producing stem cells. Breast cancer patients risk death in order to buy a chance at cure. The mistaken doses of chemotherapy at Dana-Farber tragically highlight the tension between hope for cure and the destructive potential of aggressive, potentially lifesaving therapies. If desperate women—and their physicians—are willing to take such risks, how can new therapies such as bone marrow transplant for breast cancer be evaluated? Innovative, dramatic, and lifesaving technologies hold special cultural appeal in the United States. What features of this unique social context shape the technology assessment process?

High-dose chemotherapy for breast cancer is but one of many experimental technologies that have been widely adopted for use against life-threatening illness while their safety and effectiveness are still in question. A recent press release from the National Cancer Institute begins, "Thousands of breast cancer patients are undergoing high-dose chemotherapy and bone marrow transplantation without definitive evidence that it works better than standard therapies."[2] Other examples of dramatic technologies that have been widely used prior to formal evaluation include the "gamma knife,"[3] extracorporeal membrane oxygenation,[4] and fetal neural tissue transplantation for conditions ranging from Parkinson's and Alzheimer's diseases to spinal cord injury.[5] Scientifically accepted methods of technology assessment are designed to answer questions about a new treatment's safety and effectiveness. An examination of the pathways followed by medical innovations reveals the significance of the unique social and cultural environment in which technologies are developed, evaluated, and used. The complex social context in which technological innovations in medicine are embedded—including varied local practice settings, strongly held physician and patient values, the political power of advocacy organizations, and economic or market factors—presents a challenge to formal utility assessment. Unfortunately, these potent social and cultural factors are generally excluded from consideration, as if the scientific force of "the data" could overcome their power.

Using rescue technologies for breast cancer as a case example, in this chapter we examine the social factors leading to the rapid adoption of aggressive therapeutic innovations, and the implications of these contextual factors for the conduct of technology assessment. We examine the process of assessment, both formal and informal, arguing that through these processes technologies are defined and made meaningful by various constituencies—patients, researchers, insurers—involved in their development and use. We argue that assessment of a technology, determining whether or not a treatment "works," takes place through a process of meaning construction that occurs at multiple sites. This analysis is based on 1) a review of the technical and popular literature about high-dose chemotherapy for breast cancer, 2) interviews with medical oncologists specializing in breast cancer treatment, physicians providing bone marrow transplant, breast cancer patients, insurers, and members of advocacy organizations, and 3) a focus group held at Stanford University as part of The Hastings Center technology assessment project. The focus group included transplant physicians, representatives of third-party payers, hospital administrators, nurses, health law experts, and clinicians.[6]

The field of technology assessment developed in pursuit of increasingly objective and scientific bases for clinical and policy decision making about the best use of medical technologies. The principal tool for assessing new medical technologies is the randomized controlled trial,[7] while other techniques are employed to develop objective data concerning patient preference, quality of life, and costs.[8] Nonetheless, experimental procedures frequently move into clinical practice before they have been adequately evaluated.[9] The forces behind rapid adoption of a medical technology are generally recognized to include many elements external to the technology itself or to the narrow question of whether a new treatment "works." As Banta states, "The use of technology is not merely a technical question, but is embedded in a broader framework of culture, attitudes, values, and beliefs."[10]

In spite of this recognition, the actual procedures of technology assessment do not allow for serious attention to how social and cultural context shapes the evaluation of new treatments. The factors considered to be "legitimate" in the scientific-technology assessment paradigm actually preclude serious attention to contextual features, in effect separating the technology from an entire range of social phenomena through which the technology becomes meaningful to its producers, providers, and users. Conventional technology assessment techniques frequently fail to identify the social complexities through which the issues of effectiveness, safety, superiority, and acceptability are negotiated and contested. As a result, "objective" evaluation data may lack utility and even legitimacy to practicing physicians in constant contact with desperately ill patients. The central questions addressed by technology assessment—does the technology work, how well, for whom, and at what costs?—are interwoven in the local practice setting with the lessons of clinical experience.

We argue that the construction, negotiation, and transformations of meaning that occur in technological innovation take place in a variety of social contexts and involve the local assessments of health care providers, researchers, patients, administrators, politicians, funders, drug and equipment manufacturers, and so on.[11] Technologies are evaluated within a heterogeneous web of beliefs, values, interests, and relationships that not only condition how a technology is understood, accepted, and used but also influence how effectiveness data are developed and interpreted.

High-dose chemotherapy (HDC) and autologous stem cell rescue (ASCR) by bone marrow transplantation (BMT) or peripheral blood stem cell rescue (hereafter referred to as HDC/ASCR) presents a useful case study for examining the complex social factors that affect the use and assessment of aggressive, high-cost, lifesaving technological innovations. HDC/ASCR is one of the most controversial areas of cancer treatment today. Initially used with some success for certain hematological cancers, the treatment showed promise in the treatment of women in the advanced stages of breast cancer. But treatment-related mortality and morbidity were high, and the procedure was expensive. Per procedure cost estimates generally range from $50,000 to $200,000[12] but may be as high as $380,000.[13] In spite of the treatment's high cost and high risk, use of the technique for breast cancer has become widespread and in fact now far exceeds its use for other types of cancer.[14] Many major medical centers have BMT programs that treat women with breast cancer, while private companies such as Resource Technologies also provide the treatment.

HDC/ASCR has been, and continues to be, assessed using currently accepted techniques: retrospectively through meta-analysis of available Phase I/II data and prospectively in three national randomized, controlled clinical trials in the United States. The first randomized trial comparing high-dose chemotherapy regimens with conventional chemotherapy was recently reported by a group in South Africa.[15] The results of these assessment efforts have provided support to proponents of HDC/ASCR yet failed to convince skeptics. The central medical debate concerns the relative effectiveness of high-dose chemotherapy for breast cancer compared with conventional therapies and whether high-dose therapy remains investigational or is now the standard of care for breast cancer in some circumstances. This unanswered question has significant implications, most notably for women's access to the treatment through their insurance. The emotional character of conflicts over the use of HDC/ASCR reflects the symbolic salience of aggressive, potentially lifesaving therapies in the U.S. health care system, complicating the resolution of the scientific and medical issues. How can women be denied a new treatment for breast cancer?

Local Assessment of Technologies

HDC/ASCR has become a site of multiple conflicts over meaning as varying interpretations of assessment data emerge and the technology itself changes through continuing innovation and use. Key to understanding these contestations is the process of *local assessment of technologies*. Local assessment occurs in the context of diverse social arenas that interact with the technology, including regional medical communities, professional groups, cancer patient support groups, pharmaceutical and medical-device industries, and legal and insurance entities. Issues of efficacy, safety, and acceptability are contested and negotiated. Social factors (professional ideology, local practice standards, experience with the technology, physician values and preferences, patient demand, public awareness, political interest, and cultural understandings of breast cancer) shape how the hard "facts" produced in the process of technology assessment are interpreted and used. In a sense, biomedicine has become a field where economic and political interests significantly affect technology production and utilization. Yet, as we have argued, traditional approaches to the processes of technology assessment and practice guideline development leave aside the realms of meaning and action in which these forces operate. In contrast, our analysis reveals how the local assessment of HDC/ASCR has shaped the evaluation and diffusion of the technology.

By way of background, we first present a brief overview of recent theoretical work describing how the meanings of medical practices are constructed through social processes. Next we discuss the HDC/ASCR procedure in some detail, explaining its history, scientific rationale, and impact on patients. We then turn to the social context of technological innovation and assessment through the case of HDC/ASCR, examining the sources of pressure to utilize an unproven therapy, intraprofessional variation within the medical community, the formal assessment process (including randomized clinical trials), legal issues affecting insurance coverage, and the politics of the women's health movement. We examine the conflicts and transformations in meaning that have occurred within the many groups that have been involved in the development and use of HDC/ASCR technology, looking at how social processes affect, and are affected by, formal technology assessment efforts.

The Social Context of Technology Assessment: Theoretical Perspectives

Recent work in medical sociology and anthropology has emphasized the "social construction" of biomedical knowledge. The traditional view that science represents an objective and value-free body of knowledge has been overturned in favor of an approach that recognizes that all knowledge is inherently contextual, culturally located. Margaret Lock has summarized this theoretical trend: "Our purpose is to demonstrate the social and cultural character of *all* [emphasis in original] medical knowledge, but by so doing we are not denying the existence of real, painful stress and suffering. There is, of course, a biological reality, but the moment that efforts are made to explain, order, and manipulate that reality, then a process of contextualization takes place in which the dynamic relationships of biology with cultural values and the social order has to be considered."[16] This approach opens up previously unexamined issues of objectivity in Western scientific epistemologies, including the foundational assumptions of technology assessment practices. A related trend in the interdisciplinary field of social studies of science and technology joins the study of scientific knowledge and medical practice.[17] Scholars have only recently focused on the nature of medical practice, including how scientific knowledge is incorporated into practice.[18] Medical sociologists, on the other hand, have traditionally approached subjects such as physician autonomy without critical examination of the role of scientific knowledge in clinical and investigatory work. Combining these disciplinary perspectives allows us to examine how medical practice and scientific knowledge interact as knowledges and technologies are assimilated into medical work in the forms of medical criteria, diagnostic techniques, and therapeutic options.[19]

Of course, it is also essential to look beyond the local practice context; broad social, historical, and political forces are implicated as well. For example, the use of BMT technologies to treat breast cancer has had a significant impact on the practice of clinical oncology and on the conduct of clinical research in breast cancer and perhaps other areas. Trends include the shifting relationships of power and influence among researchers, clinicians, insurers, and both state and federal policy entities.

Theoretical focus on the articulation of scientific knowledge and medical practice raises a number of questions that are germane to the technology evaluation process. What are the implications, for clinical practice and the development of new scientific knowledge, of their constant coupling in the context of clinical research? How is closure reached on scientific inquiry in the practice setting? In medical practice, decisions must be made for a particular patient in spite of the uncertain and evolving nature of scientific knowledge; what are the implications, for scientific and clinical activities, of differing imperatives? How are the economic impacts of innovations defined, measured, and interpreted, and what effects do these interpretations have on practice?

What happens to scientific knowledge and novel technologies as they come into contact with patients in medical practice? Patients are at once objects of medical technologies and subjects of their treatment experiences. That patients are subjective, embodied actors whose experiences in medical practice reflect powerfully back into the constitution of knowledge and practice is perhaps most significant in the context of experimental therapies.[20] The process of treatment innovation is continually altered by actions and understandings of the "socio-political bodies" of patients/subjects.[21]

Recent work in "technoscience studies" has also expanded our view of technological objects.[22] Rather than being viewed as bounded and stable entities, technologies are seen as bundles of knowledge, practice, and artifact that are continually shifting as problems are solved and as demands of the specific practice context and larger social order are met. In the process of biomedical innovation, complex, high-risk experimental therapies such as HDC/ASCR are constantly reconfigured as data from their use is fed back into the innovation process. Reconfiguration and innovation also occur in local practice sites as technologies are adapted to unique clinical circumstances. The data about experimental therapies gathered from local practice settings include not only the "hard facts" of blood counts, ejection fractions, and lab results but unique

132   Part II: Outcomes Data

information produced through social interaction. The production of this local knowledge is influenced by many factors, including commercial interests in capturing a market for a particular machine, local and/or societal concerns about cost and risk, insurance reimbursement decisions, oversupply or lack of trained technical support, research agendas of colleagues and referring physicians, patient population characteristics, and location and quality of lab facilities. Technologies, then, are continually being configured, negotiated, and assessed both locally and in interaction with broader (professional, legal, political, financial, and scientific) factors. They are "moving targets" of evaluation efforts. Technologies are not simply "given"—their form and nature are continually renegotiated and their status reinterpreted over time.

The Case Study: High-Dose Chemotherapy of Breast Cancer followed by Autologous Bone Marrow Transplantation and/or Peripheral Stem Cell Rescue

According to the American Cancer Society,[23] an estimated 180,200 women will develop breast cancer in 1997, and 43,900 will die of the disease. Most new cases of breast cancer are diagnosed in women with localized and regional disease, while only 5–10 percent of patients present with metastatic disease.[24] Adjuvant (low-dose) chemotherapy has been considered the standard treatment for most women with nonmetastatic breast cancer at least since the mid-1980s,[25] and significant improvements in disease-free and overall survival have been achieved.[26] Metastatic breast cancer, however, is widely believed to be incurable, with a median survival of only two years. Most women who are diagnosed with metastatic breast cancer will die of their disease in a relatively short time.[27]

Chemotherapeutic drugs at "low" or conventional doses often fail to kill the stray malignant cells that eventually result in metastases. The concept of dose response in chemotherapy has provided the rationale for high-dose therapies: alkylating agents (a type of chemotherapy) exhibit a steep, logarithmic curve in their cancer-killing effect.[28] But the patient's hematopoietic system—bone marrow, white and red blood cells, platelets, and stem cells—is destroyed in the process, leaving the patient unable to fight infection or stop bleeding. Bone marrow transplantation procedures developed thirty years ago make it possible to regenerate blood cells and reconstitute the immune system so that chemotherapy can be given at extremely high, once deadly levels.[29]

Prior to the development of bone marrow transplantation techniques, destruction of the hematopoietic system was defined as the primary factor limiting dose levels of chemotherapeutic drugs. With high-dose chemotherapy, upper dose limits are now defined by damage in other organs: the kidney, liver, heart, and lungs. High-dose regimens involve many times the standard dose. For example, the standard dose of the drug ifosfamide is 5,000 mg/m^2, while the high dose used is 18,000 mg/m^2.[30] The severe toxicities produced by high-dose chemotherapy make the process a grueling and dangerous one. "Early death" (defined as mortality from treatment-related complications within thirty days of stem cell rescue) has continued to be a problem, occurring in 10–20 percent of patients reported in recent trials.[31]

As recently as twenty years ago, bone marrow transplantation was strictly an investigational procedure.[32] Donor, or allogeneic, bone marrow transplantation is now recognized as an effective treatment for "diffuse" cancers such as certain leukemias, Hodgkin's disease, and non-Hodgkin's lymphomas. Use of this procedure is limited by the difficulty of finding immunologically compatible donors to reduce the possibility of rejection. Development of procedures for harvesting, storing, and reinfusing a patient's own bone marrow (autologous transplantation) raised the potential of high-dose chemotherapy for treating the more common solid tumors, including breast, ovarian, and testicular cancers and childhood neuroblastomas. These cancers respond to, but are not cured by, chemotherapy. A more recent innovation has been the use of autologous peripheral blood stem cell rescue, in which stem cells are removed from the patient's circulating blood and reinfused after high-dose chemotherapy. The use of hematopoietic growth factors, drugs that stimulate stem cell production before harvesting and to speed engraftment following reinfusion, has been a further refinement of the procedure.

The Autologous Blood and Marrow Transplant Registry—North America has reported that, between 1989 and 1992, the major indication in the United States and Canada for HDC/ASCR changed from non-Hodgkin's lymphoma to breast cancer.[33] In Europe, use of the procedure for solid tumors, including breast cancer, appears to have lagged behind that in North America, constituting only about 8 percent of European HDC/ASCR cases in 1992.[34]

The HDC/ASCR procedure continues to evolve, both in terms of the technologies employed and the patient populations to which they are applied. The procedure typically involves the following steps: pretreatment, stem cell harvesting, stem cell processing and storage, administration of high-dose chemotherapy, reinfusion of stem cells, and hematopoietic recovery.[35] Some centers perform "tandem" or sequential rounds of HDC/ASCR.[36] These general steps are performed in a number of ways, leading to much local practice variation in what is generally referred to as HDC/ASCR. For example, studies reported in the literature have used different patient selection criteria and different combinations of drugs at different doses in both the pretreatment (or "induction") and high-dose phases of the treatment. Different regimens are constantly being tried in small, uncontrolled Phase I/II studies. Many elements of the procedure are in constant flux, as demonstrated by Vaughan.[37] The features of constant transformation, idiosyncratic regimens and supporting rationale, and confusion concerning the therapy's status for different uses (e.g., "investigational," "reasonable therapeutic option," "standard therapy") have contributed significantly to the ways in which formal and informal technology assessments have proceeded.

Patients must meet certain physical criteria before they are considered candidates for HDC/ASCR. A review of published studies has shown that metastatic women aged sixty-five or younger whose central nervous system, liver, kidney, and cardiopulmonary functions were not damaged met the basic selection criteria. Many studies used minimal disease (lower tumor burden) as the major criteria.[38] Usually, patients must have disease that responds to chemotherapy. It is difficult to determine patient selection criteria for the majority of HDC/ASCR procedures because they are performed outside of clinical trial settings.[39]

After stem cell harvesting, patients are treated with high doses of chemotherapy, usually in combinations of two or three drugs.[40] The drugs may be given over the course of two to six days. Patients may also undergo radiation therapy. The high-dose regimen leaves the patient highly susceptible to infections. Patients may be confined to isolation in a specially designed laminar airflow room (equipped with high efficiency particulate air filters to reduce the risk of infection). Stem cells are usually reinfused within twenty-four to seventy-two hours after chemotherapy is administered—this is the "rescue" process.

Patients remain susceptible to a number of disorders and infections for up to six months after transplantation, including bacterial, fungal, viral, or parasitic infections and pulmonary infiltrates, dermatitis, cystitis, bleeding, diarrhea, mouth soreness, and other gastrointestinal problems.[41] Supportive care during this period is focused on the prevention of infection and the management of side effects, including anemia, bleeding, nausea, vomiting, loss of appetite, and malfunction of the lungs, liver, kidneys, and heart. Patients therefore receive a variety of ancillary therapies. For example, because damage to the gastrointestinal tract can be severe, some patients are unable to eat for several months and are instead supported with total parenteral nutrition.

Following discharge, patients may need to retain a vascular-access catheter for future administration of blood products to treat anemia and thrombocytopenia. Follow-up visits to the transplant center continue frequently for several months, then less frequently based on each patient's need. Most follow-up includes bone marrow aspiration to monitor the condition of the marrow. Many patients need a year or more to recover physically and psychologically—even then, life may never return to "normal." Patients we interviewed reported increased fatigue and the need for constant vigilance against "overdoing it."[42] The procedure can cause great stress for the patients and their families, who must often struggle with the financial aspects of the treatment as well as the other disruptions in their lives.[43] And in spite of the extreme lengths to which they have gone to battle their cancer, many women still suffer from constant fear of remission, described by one woman as the "ax hanging over our heads."

Examining the Social Context: HDC/ASCR for Breast Cancer

In the early clinical investigation of HDC for breast cancer, social factors shaped how the technology entered medical practice, how technology assessment data were developed, and the "failure" of efforts to control the technology. These contextual factors included features of medical practice and clinical research, ideologies of biomedicine and cancer, features of the patient population, as well as institutional, financial, and legal considerations.

Several factors were key to the rapid adoption of HDC/ASCR for breast cancer. First, there were few structural barriers to the use of the HDC/ASCR procedure. This is in contrast to novel pharmaceuticals or medical devices that are carefully regulated by the Food and Drug Administration. Chemotherapy drugs are readily available; physicians and hospitals, particularly those already offering bone marrow transplantation for other illnesses, were able to begin offering and refining the treatment, using existing tools and resources. Resistance from third-party payers based on cost concerns proved to be the greatest obstacle to diffusion of HDC/ASCR therapy for breast cancer. Second, the moral imperatives to try the new therapy were strong. Initial experiences with HDC for breast cancer showed "promise"; according to some enthusiasts, the promise included a cure for metastatic disease. With little else to offer their patients and with strong motivation to pursue whatever treatment might offer hope, many physicians and patients pushed for access to the treatment. They were supported by the tenacious structural and ideological forces pursuing the goal of a cancer cure.[44] Third, the proliferation of small, uncontrolled studies of inconsistent quality[45] provided ambiguous assessment data that could be employed to support conflicting claims about the efficacy of HDC/ASCR. Contradictions, ambiguities, and inconsistencies in the scientific literature—the primary reporting mechanism for formal assessment data—facilitated use of the data to support conflicting claims about the technology. Gathering definitive evidence has been difficult. Many doctors, already convinced that "more chemotherapy is better," have offered HDC/ASCR to women outside clinical trials, impeding accrual to NCI-sponsored research.[46] Such actions are justified with moral claims; physicians express concern about depriving patients of the treatment's benefit.

When researchers initially began to assess the feasibility of using the high-dose chemotherapy technologies employed in the treatment of diffuse cancer for treating solid-tumor cancers, it was in the context of "salvage" therapy for breast cancer patients with advanced disease who were not responding to conventional treatment. Early Phase I trials with metastatic breast cancer patients who had previously undergone intensive chemotherapy treatment were encouraging.[47] These trials involved only a small number of patients. Many of these patients had refractory disease, that is, cancer that did not respond to prior chemotherapy. A partial remission of short duration (median duration range from these studies was 2–5 months) was achieved in 56–75 percent of the patients,[48] including some of those with refractory cancer. But the incidence of fatal complications—such as bacterial or fungal infection, liver disease, or cardiac damage—was high.

The achievement of some apparent success with metastatic patients gave rise to considerable excitement among researchers and patients. Phase II studies were continued with women with metastatic disease.[49] The populations enrolled in these studies were diverse, including patients who had just become Stage IV, had not previously undergone intensive chemotherapy treatment, or were in their first relapse after remission. These trials tested various chemotherapeutic agents and achieved a significant decline in treatment-related deaths due to better infection control procedures and the use of growth colony–stimulating factors and peripheral stem cells to speed the engraftment of bone marrow and recovery of the immune system. All agreed that HDC is highly toxic,[50] but there was little consensus in the medical community about the interpretation of results of these studies. Although reviews of the scientific literature began to appear in the late 1980s, they could not conclude that HDC/ASCR offered a significant benefit above conventional treatment for women with metastatic disease. During the 1980s, the results were sufficiently ambiguous to support both the enthusiasm of transplant proponents and the skepticism of critics.

The greater tumor burden of patients with metastatic disease appeared to be a limiting factor in use of HDC for advanced disease, an issue that had been raised by Armitage much earlier.[51] Many researchers have found the procedure to be too risky for women over the age of sixty-five. Transplant investigators have more recently studied the use of HDC/ASCR in woman with early-stage, high-risk breast cancer.[52] These patients tend to be younger and to have less extensive cancers. Trials are being designed to determine when chemotherapy followed by HDC/ASCR will improve survival rates of Stage II breast cancer patients whose cancer has spread to lymph nodes under the arms, and Stage III patients who are in a first remission and have not yet relapsed but are at high risk for relapse. Exploration also is beginning into the effectiveness of HDC/ASCR for treating women with inflammatory or locally unresectable breast cancer.[53]

Social and Cultural Sources of Pressure to Utilize an "Unproven Therapy"

While much of the urgency for defining the role of HDC/ASCR in the treatment of breast cancer derived from pressures in insurance, legal, and patient advocacy arenas, the procedure remains controversial within the medical community. Central to the controversy has been the appropriate interpretation of a situation of uncertainty: emergent, ambiguous data concerning the efficacy and safety of high-dose chemotherapy, the patient populations most likely to receive benefit, and role of high-dose chemotherapy among current and novel treatment options available to patients. They have also involved issues that are more clearly normative. Do patients have the right to demand unproven treatments? Do insurers have the right to deny them access? Is offering a patient an unproven, expensive treatment an acceptable use of medical resources? How should the costs of clinical research be distributed?[54] We argue that interpretation of uncertainty in medical practice is guided by the "tenacious" background assumptions and practices of biomedical culture[55] within the framework of local practice experience and pressures.

The first background assumption framing interpretive responses to ambiguous and uncertain data—such as data about the usefulness of HDC/ASCR—derives from the epistemological stance of naturalism.[56] This stance sustains the belief that an objective and definitive answer to questions of a technology's efficacy is possible and inevitable, given the appropriate scientific methods of inquiry. As stated on August 11, 1994, by Bruce Cheson of the National Cancer Institute (NCI) before a subcommittee hearing on federal-employee health care benefits and breast cancer:

> The NCI believes that clinical trials of ABMT for the treatment of patients with tumors such as breast cancer are essential to determine the safety and efficacy of this procedure. Only through the conduct of well-designed prospective studies can we determine if this approach is of benefit, including the specific diseases and specific patient groups for which it is appropriate. Currently, NCI sponsored clinical trials are carefully addressing

138 Part II: Outcomes Data

these important issues. For patients with breast cancer, more data are needed to definitively establish the role of ABMT as standard therapy in these disease settings. . . . We believe that routine use in clinical practice should occur only after scientific evaluation establishes its value. [Bruce Cheson, *Congressional Testimony before the Subcommittee on Compensation Employee Benefits, Committee on Post Office and Civil Service: Autologous Bone Marrow Transplantation as a Treatment for Breast Cancer*, Federal Document Clearing House, August 11, 1994.]

Implicit in this interpretive framework is a model of progress and perfectibility in science: an ethos upon which the war on cancer and its associated medical practices, institutions, and political, economic, and personal investments have been built.[57] Although some novel cancer drugs and regimens have been developed, and progress made in cancers such as Hodgkin's disease and testicular carcinoma, many patients still die from their disease or from the consequences of treatment.[58] New therapies are frequently surrounded with an aura of progressive optimism, a persistent hope that continued technological advance will result in the ability to produce long-term cures. Dramatic results such as those reported in some early, small studies of HDC/ASCR for breast cancer, when placed in the context of the relative failure of conventional therapies, both illustrate and fuel the progressive ideology. According to Smith and Henderson, "[T]he rapid growth of HDC/ABMT technology since the early 1980s was based on the premise that therapy of breast cancer is not palliative, *but instead can provide a long-term cure* [emphasis added]."[59]

The second background assumption framing or sustaining practitioners' interpretations and judgments about the value of a new technology reflects the Western tradition of individualism—"a complex of values and assumptions asserting the primacy of the individual and of individual freedom."[60] Individualism is embodied by autonomous, proactive, and "free" agents. This vision of agency is reflected in many models of clinical, research, and even patient orientation to medical technologies. In the case of HDC/ASCR, both researchers and patients have portrayed themselves, and been widely portrayed in media accounts and patient-oriented literatures, as innovators, rule-breaking pioneers, and heroes. The efforts of some patients to obtain access to HDC/ASCR also reflect the ethos of individualism, expressed in a belief that they are being denied access to something to which they have a natural right.[61]

Traditions in clinical practice are also influenced by individualism, in particular the ethos of "working for your patient against the rules." For example, an active transplant physician reported engaging in "rule breaking" in order to circumvent insurer restrictions on HDC/ASCR; high-dose chemotherapy was administered on an outpatient basis, and patients admitted to the hospital only when they "crashed." The objective of this practice was to break the treatment down into standard reimbursement units that would not raise questions about experimental therapy. Many innovations in the procedure were similarly aimed at reducing costs and increasing the likelihood of insurance reimbursement. For example, researchers at Duke pioneered the use of isolated stays in hotel rooms rather than in the traditional sterile laminar flow rooms for patients during the period of greatest vulnerability to viral or fungal infection.

Intraprofessional Variation and Local Assessments of HDC/ABMT Data

Armstrong has pointed out that the increasing development of guidelines for patient care, emerging from the development of clinical scientific knowledge, challenges the personal authority of a physician's individual expertise.[62] Further, not all physicians are connected with the research activities, primarily clinical trials, that form the technology assessment process for innovations such as HDC/ASCR. While some physicians are actively involved in the development and application of bone marrow transplantation therapies—working in or building transplant centers, obtaining research grants, publishing data, and employing novel techniques—other physicians interact more sporadically with transplantation as one among a range of treatment options (including other novel therapies). Not all physicians accept that Autologous Bone Marrow Transplantation should have a central role in treating breast cancer; intraprofessional variation[63] is, not surprisingly, reflected in the manner in which evaluative data are interpreted. Perspectives vary according to medical specialty and participation in research.

Bone marrow transplant physicians we interviewed fit the model of "experimenters" put forward by sociologist Anselm Strauss and colleagues.[64] Experimenters define their "core task as generating scientific data by placing their eligible patients into experimental programs."[65] Transplanters, like experimenters, tend to view HDC/ASCR in terms of a continuum of innovation. In the continuum model the process of therapeutic innovation progresses from animal studies, to small clinical studies with terminally ill patients beyond the scope of conventional therapies, to less critically ill patients in randomized studies that compare innovations to the optimum standard treatment. This view mirrors the progress of HDC/ASCR innovation for breast cancer, from "salvage" therapy in women with advanced metastatic disease, to clinical trials as first-line adjuvant therapy for women with high-risk disease, to randomized clinical trials comparing high-dose therapies with similar conventional-dose regimens in metastatic and high-risk women. To physicians active in bone marrow transplantation, extension of HDC/ASCR from diffuse cancers to solid tumors such as breast cancer has been a logical, inevitable, and progressive step in the battle against cancer. It is yet another disease against which their technology can be employed and, for academic physicians, another way to advance one's career.[66]

Transplant proponents are optimists. They are able to see beyond high morbidity and mortality—caused by infections and toxicity—to the improvements in the treatment achieved by refinements, such as the use of growth-stimulating factors and peripheral stem cells, and to the increasing ability to manage complications. In contrast, medical oncologists—"therapists," according to Strauss's categorization[67]—define their primary responsibility in terms of the particular patient. Each therapeutic innovation is but one of a range of available alternatives. For active clinicians the emphasis is on the routine application of standard therapy. The blend of situated experience, intuition, and local knowledge comprising the "practical expertise" behind clinical decision making forms a significance aspect of their interpretation of technology assessment data.

Formal Assessments of HDC/ASCR

The regional structure of clinical trial groups supported by the NCI disseminates innovations beyond a few major clinical sites.[68] Many physicians, however, have begun providing or referring their patients for bone marrow transplantation outside the randomized clinical trials rather than risk randomization to the control, or "conventional" therapy arm, of a trial.[69] Women, using a variety of informational resources, also seek out and travel to centers that perform the procedure.

While the NCI-sponsored Phase III clinical trials have not been completed at this writing, the scientific literature on HDC/ASCR for breast cancer contains a number of attempts to review clinical and investigatory experience with the procedure.[70] While all of the reviews agree that further evidence from randomized, controlled clinical trials is necessary to determine whether HDC/ASCR is superior to conventional therapy for high-risk or metastatic disease, they reach different conclusions regarding currently available data. Some investigators are clearly convinced that further refinement will make this the treatment of choice for select patients; others await the outcomes of the NCI-sponsored national randomized clinical trials with the implication that they will provide clear answers from which practice guidelines will be developed. The quality of existing and emergent assessment data, and interpretations drawn from them, have been continuing points of contestation.

Legal Pressures and the Insurance Industry Response

Disputes about whether HDC/ASCR for metastatic or early breast cancer are experimental or "standard of care" have had enormous visibility—and impact—in the legal and health care–financing arenas. Legal battles waged between breast cancer patients and their insurers—including reports of large settlements—have been reported in the major media,[71] fueling public sentiment against insurers as well as interest in the treatment. Researchers, academic and community cancer centers, and other providers have a great interest in seeing HDC/ASCR recognized as a nonexperimental, medically necessary treatment for breast cancer in some circumstances. Likewise, they have strong interest in promoting the involvement of third-party payers in funding clinical research.[72] The issue of what meanings are assigned to technology, in what circumstances, and by whom has become critically important in the process of financing medical innovation and treatment. Because multiple domains of action and interest are involved, conflicts occur when meaning is imported from one domain to another. For example, a clinician may produce abundant evidence in her case to the insurance company that HDC/ASCR is the accepted treatment for her patient's diagnosis and, at the same time require the patient to give informed consent in order to receive an experimental procedure. This type of domain conflict produced a number of "workarounds" or innovations in the system that served to facilitate the acceptance and use of HDC/ASCR. We will focus on the following issues in examining contested issues in the legal and financial arena of HDC/ASCR for breast cancer: negotiation and debate about the experimental nature of bone marrow transplantation, the development of legal resources and strategies to influence insurance company decisions, and debates about the appropriate distribution of clinical-trial costs.

According to the *Bone Marrow Transplant Newsletter*,[73] more than 200 people were unable to undergo a bone marrow transplant between 1988 and 1991 because their insurance company would not cover the cost of the procedure. The newsletter's survey data indicated that autologous bone marrow transplantation is the type most frequently resisted by insurance companies, particularly if the treatment is for breast cancer or other solid tumors. Experience with claims denial by Peters and Rogers[74] at the Duke University Bone Marrow Transplantation Program showed the preauthorization process of private and employer-based insurers to be "arbitrary and capricious" for women with breast cancer. And in spite of the numerous technology reviews conducted by major health insurers,[75] data from the Duke program showed that patients with advanced metastatic breast cancer who were enrolled in dose-finding Phase I trials were approved as often as were patients enrolled in multicenter randomized trials given a high priority by the National Cancer Institute (86 percent vs. 90 percent).[76] The implication is that denials were not based on the amount of evidence or level of acceptability within the cancer research community concerning HDC/ASCR for different applications but, rather, on political pressure or case-by-case assessments relying on other factors. One transplant nurse we interviewed described a typical workaround: an early HDC/ABMT recipient from her hospital—an attorney—was enlisted to aid later patients in developing effective strategies for pressuring insurance companies. This example illustrates the important role of patients.

The majority of insurance claim denials and subsequent legal battles were not about the particulars of the treatment per se but over contractual language excluding payment for experimental treatments, a long-standing industry practice. Pressure to change these practices began as a response to the demand for emerging therapies by AIDS patients in the 1980s. The similarity of issues in insurance coverage for experimental treatments for AIDS and breast cancer allowed an easy translation of legal strategies used against the insurers. The territory was familiar, the groundwork laid. As one attorney experienced in both areas described the relationship, "It took about five minutes to set up a panel to handle breast cancer issues, and it took years to set up an AIDS referral panel."

Political influence has also been pivotal to the process of acceptance and diffusion of HDC/ASCR for breast cancer. In 1994, largely in response to enormous political pressure, the Office of Personnel Management issued an order mandating that all 350 health plans serving nine million federal employees and dependents cover HDC/ASCR treatments for breast cancer.

In the context of legal, financial, and political struggles over HDC/ASCR, the lack of solid evidence allowed multiple interpretations of the procedure to be put forward credibly. Interpretations of the technology were presented to support positions that were strongly influenced by emotions, professional self-interest, and political pressures. The trend toward coverage by various forms of insurance and the persistence and increasing success of litigation created a momentum for diffusion of the technology beyond clinical trials at major academic centers. It became—from the perspective of insurers—more difficult *not* to cover the procedure than to cover it. Bear in mind that this occurs whether or not the treatment "works."

While the interpretation of HDC/ASCR as experimental or standard of care for breast cancer was in flux, the relationship between the insurance industry and research funding became unstable. By demanding coverage of a treatment still under evaluation, patients and researchers forced insurers to reexamine their role in research. Where insurers traditionally had waited until a standard had been agreed upon within the medical community before extending coverage to a novel treatment, they were now participating in the evaluation process by funding their patients' participation in clinical trials. The traditional research "partnership" between clinical researchers and patients is transformed; they are now joined by industry, government, consumer groups, and third-party payers.

Political Bodies: Breast Cancer and the Social Context of Women's Health

Bone marrow transplant for breast cancer evolved simultaneously with pressure from a variety of sources to increase funding for women's health and bring women's concerns to the forefront of the federal research agenda. Legislative activities in the 1990s created the Women's Health Equity Act, which in 1993 authorized the Office of Research on Women's Health within the NIH. In 1991, NIH director Bernadine Healy announced plans for the Women's Health Initiative, a major longitudinal study of preventive mechanisms for osteoporosis, cancer, and cardiovascular disease in postmenopausal women.[77] Breast cancer is one of the major foci of the new policy attention to women's health, as evidenced by significant increases in funding for breast cancer research and the implementation of the National Breast Cancer Action Plan under the office of the deputy assistant secretary for women's health.

Women's success at controlling the national medical-research agenda followed from the successes of AIDS activists in increasing funding for AIDS research, expanding access to experimental therapies, and incorporating consumer participation in evaluation of technology assessment data. During the placebo-controlled trials of AZT—then the only treatment offering a possibility of benefit—AIDS activists forcefully argued that participation in clinical trials was a benefit to which wider access should be made available. Political pressures yielded changes in the federal regulatory process for the development and licensing of new drugs, allowing "expanded access," participation in "parallel track" studies, and easier access to investigational drugs through investigational new drug (IND) protocols. Levine argues that during this era the public's understanding of participation in a clinical trial changed significantly, from a potentially dangerous situation in which one could be exposed to an experimental drug or procedure, to the only means of access to a "promising new therapy."[78]

Breast cancer advocacy groups such as the National Breast Cancer Coalition have successfully raised the level of public awareness about the disease and have gained considerable legislative support for their agenda of increased federal efforts to improve breast cancer treatment. Through a variety of mechanisms and largely working with the National Cancer Institute and other members of the "cancer establishment," advocates have encouraged breast cancer patients to educate themselves regarding their treatment options. Conventional treatments for these cancers are disappointing and take a severe toll on a woman's body. Many women with breast cancer, their physicians, and their supporters are actively searching for treatments that are superior to conventional therapy, particularly for high-risk and metastatic cancers. The high visibility of breast cancer on the national agenda—particularly the widespread impatience with scientific progress to date—is in itself a potent background force shaping efforts to evaluate HDC/ASCR.

Everyone waits for the good news to break. An effective popularizing mechanism for HDC/ASCR treatment has been the telling of "heroic stories." An article in the *Bone Marrow Transplant Newsletter* begins, "Laura Evans, someone you should know." Ms. Evans, a young woman who underwent a grueling treatment of high-dose chemotherapy and bone marrow transplantation for breast cancer, resolved to return posttherapy to her passionate involvement with mountain climbing. Her quest evolved into a well-publicized climb described in an advertisement for Bristol-Myers Squibb: "Don't Tell Them It's Insurmountable. As breast cancer survivors, these determined women have conquered mountains more intimidating than Aconcagua, even though it's one of the largest in the Western Hemisphere—they've conquered mountains of their own. That's why this expedition recently scaled Mt. Aconcagua to raise breast health awareness and funds for the fight against breast cancer—hoping that each step they took would bring them one more step closer to a cure."

Women making decisions about breast cancer treatments are faced with uncertainty and ambiguity. Women we interviewed relied on two major sources of information and advice in making decisions about HDC therapy—their primary physician (generally their oncologist or general surgeon) and the support groups in which they participate. Support groups serve as local sites of anecdotal-information exchange as well as forums for the circulation of data from the popular and scientific literatures. Women exchange stories and information about their own treatment experiences and seek comparable elements of their stories ("another women whose tumor didn't show up on mammogram"). In small information networks, local assessments are colored by the experiences resident in that group.

When researching information about HDC/ASCR from sources beyond their local networks, women face further complications caused by the variety of HDC regimens in use at different institutions[79] and the variety of single institution–based statistics offered. A young woman was quoted in the *New York Times* as saying, "This is the hardest decision of my life. . . . I wish there was just one god of all cancers who would say, 'This is what you have to do.' But it's not working out that way."[80]

Conclusions: The Contested Meanings of HDC/ASCR

We have argued that the evaluation of novel, aggressive, and potentially lifesaving medical technologies presents serious challenges to conventional technology assessment practices. A risk worth taking, a potential cure, a possible lawsuit—multiple meanings permeate the use of HDC/ASCR for breast cancer. Like many other dramatic treatments, HDC/ASCR was widely used prior to formal evaluation efforts. Through a fundamentally *social* process of local assessment by clinicians and patients, the meaning of HDC/ASCR as a "promising new therapy" was established. Local assessments contribute to, and are influenced by, broader cultural, political, legal, economic, and social disputes over the nature and role of technologies in practice.

Boundaries between experiment and therapy are unstable. Therapies used in clinical practice are not fixed but are moving targets, rarely pierced by our efforts to evaluate them. Thus, efforts to interpret and apply outcomes data are necessarily made in a context of uncertainty. In the case of HDC/ASCR as a treatment for breast cancer, efforts for technology assessment provided data that were interpreted as either "promising" or "inconclusive," "dangerous" or "safe," depending upon the social location of the interpreter. The resulting disputes in different social arenas over the meaning of the technology shaped the process of evaluating treatment outcomes and influenced the rate of acceptance and use of HDC/ASCR.

The story of high-dose chemotherapy followed by rescue also reveals the importance of analyzing each new technology within its unique social and historical context. One source of political pressure to use the treatment came from the U.S. women's health movement, which highlighted breast cancer as a neglected disease in need of immediate attention, raising public awareness and expectations. Timing was also a crucial factor. Barriers to experimental therapies and participation in clinical trials had been torn down by a generation of AIDS activists.

The process of technology assessment in Western biomedicine is shaped by cultural beliefs in unending medical progress as well as in the sovereignty of the proactive, autonomous agent. Risky or marginal treatments may readily be framed as "promising breakthroughs," and the patients and providers who use them as courageous "heroes" and "rule breakers" who have a right to ask for or offer potentially lifesaving treatments. Cultural assumptions inform all phases of the technology assessment process. Efforts to achieve objective, scientific data about a treatment's effectiveness rest on a belief that methods such as the randomized controlled clinical trial will produce a nonambiguous and nonrefutable outcome. We have shown not only the importance of social context to the interpretation and acceptance of outcomes data but that social, political, and cultural factors are significant forces in the process of producing technology assessments. Standard models of technology assessment cannot take account of social context, of the insight that the meanings of new technologies are locally produced and shaped in interaction with cultural forces. Until this conceptual barrier is overcome, those who produce formal, objective technology assessment reports—no matter how good the data—will be left wondering why no one is listening.

NOTES

1. Lawrence K. Altman, "Big Doses of Chemotherapy Drug Killed Patient, Hurt 2d," The *New York Times*, Late Edition—Final Correction Appended Friday, March 24, 1995. Sec: A, National Desk p:18.

2. National Cancer Institute, press release, May 28, 1996.

3. Jane E. Brody, " 'Knife' Transforms Brain Surgery," *New York Times* (July 5, 1995): B6.

4. Stephen J. Elliott, "Neonatal Extracorporeal Membrane Oxygenation: How Not to Assess Novel Technologies," *Lancet* 337 (1991): 476–7.

5. Susan E. Kelly, "Moral Boundaries of Medical Research: A Sociological Analysis of Human Fetal Tissue Transplantation Research" (Ph.D. dissertation, University of California, San Francisco, 1994).

6. Initial fieldwork also included a site visit to a major academic bone marrow transplantation center during which presentations were made by providers of BMT technologies. In addition to formal interviews, many informal discussions were held with oncologists, transplant specialists, patients, breast cancer activists, and insurance attorneys to understand differing perspectives and experiences with BMT. We made use of information available to these communities:

MEDLINE searches for recent articles in the scientific literature; LEXIS/NEXIS searches for information on BMT-related legal actions; media sources, including major national and local newspapers; and sources available to breast cancer patients, including PDQ (the cancer information database developed by the National Cancer Institute), the Cancer Information Service (1-800-4-CANCER), the *BMT Newsletter*, accessed through the on-line service NYSERNet and available over the World Wide Web, InfoTrac Health Reference Center, and newsletters and other materials produced by transplant centers and breast cancer activist and support groups.

7. Clinical trials, the "gold standard" of technology assessment, may function not only to generate scientific knowledge and refine clinical practice but, ironically, to increase demand for HDC/ASCR among breast cancer patients. Barbara Koenig, "The Technological Imperative," in Margaret Lock and Deborah Gordon, eds. *Biomedicine Examined* (Dordrecht; Netherlands: Kluwer Academic Publishers) 465–96.

8. Victor R. Fuchs and Alan M. Garber, "The New Technology Assessment," *New England Journal of Medicine* 323 (1990): 673–7.

9. Ann L. Greer, "Advances in the Study of Diffusion of Innovation in Health Care," *Milbank Memorial Fund Quarterly* 55 (1977): 505–32; David H. Banta, "Social Science Research on Medical Technology: Utility and Limitations," *Social Science and Medicine* 17 (1983): 1363–9.

10. Banta, "Social Science Research," p. 1363.

11. "Local" refers both to physical and social proximity, as in the case of local practice patterns or local support groups, and to similarity in orientation and experience.

12. Bruce E. Hillner, Thomas J. Smith, and Christopher Desch, "Efficacy and Cost-Effectiveness of Autologous Bone Marrow Transplantation in Metastatic Breast Cancer: Estimates Using Decision Analysis While Awaiting Clinical Trial Results," *Journal of the American Medical Association* 267, no. 15 (1992): 2055–62.

13. ECRI, Health Technology Assessment Information Service, "High-dose Chemotherapy with Autologous Bone Marrow Transplantation and/or Blood Cell Transplantation for the Treatment of Metastatic Breast Cancer," *Executive Briefings* (February 1995): 1–12.

14. *Bone Marrow Transplants: A Book of Basics for Patients*, reprinted by NYSERNet, Inc., with permission from *BMT Newsletter* (1994).

15. W. R. Bezwoda, L. Seymour, and R. D. Dansey, "High-Dose Chemotherapy with Hematopoietic Rescue as Primary Treatment for Metastatic Breast Cancer: A Randomized Trial," *Journal of Clinical Oncology* 13 (1995): 2483–9; M. John Kennedy, "High-Dose Chemotherapy for Breast Cancer: Is the Question Answered?" *Journal of Clinical Oncology* 13 (1995): 2477–9.

16. Margaret Lock, "Introduction," in Margaret Lock and Deborah Gordon, eds., *Biomedicine Examined* (Dordrecht, Netherlands: Kluwer Academic Publishers, 1988), p. 7.

17. Monica J. Casper and Marc Berg, "Introduction: Constructivist Perspectives on Medical Practices," *Science, Technology, and Human Values* 20, no. 4 (1995): 395–407.

18. Joan H. Fujimura, "Constructing 'Do-Able' Problems in Cancer Research: Articulating Alignment," *Social Studies of Science* 17 (1987): 257–93; Joan H. Fujimura, "The Molecular Biological Bandwagon in Cancer Research: Where Social Worlds Meet," *Social Problems* 35 (1988): 261–83; Barbara A. Koenig, "The Technological Imperative in Medical Practice: The Social Construction of a 'Routine' Treatment," in Lock and Gordon, *Biomedicine Examined,* pp. 79–92; Susan L. Star, *Regions of the Mind: Brain Research and the Quest for Scientific Certainty* (Stanford: Stanford University Press, 1989).

19. Casper and Berg, "Introduction."

20. Renee C. Fox, *Experiment Perilous: Physicians and Patients Facing the Unknown* (Philadelphia: University of Pennsylvania Press, 1959).

21. Jeffrey Levi, "Unproven AIDS Therapies: The Food and Drug Administration and ddI," in Kathi E. Hanna, ed., *Biomedical Politics* (Washington, D.C.: National Academy Press, 1991), pp. 9–37; Steven Epstein, "The Construction of Lay Expertise: AIDS Activism and the Forging of Credibility in the Reform of Clinical Trials," *Science, Technology, and Human Values* 20 no. 4 (1995): 408–37.

22. Barbara A. Koenig and Monica J. Casper, "Biomedical Technologies: Reconfiguring Nature and Culture," *Medical Anthropology Quarterly* (special issue, 1996, in press).

23. American Cancer Society, *Cancer Facts and Figures* 1997 (Atlanta: American Cancer Society, 1994).

24. Metastatic (Stage IV) breast cancer is defined as the occurrence of a primary tumor of any size with ancillary lymph node involvement and distant metastases into visceral organs, bone, or the central nervous system (O.H. Beahrs et al., *Manual for Staging of Cancer,* 3rd edition, American Joint Committee on Cancer [Philadelphia: Lippincott, 1988], pp. 145–50).

25. Susan E. Myers and Stephanie F. Williams, "Role of High-Dose Chemotherapy and Autologous Stem Cell Support in Treatment of Breast Cancer," *Hematology/Oncology Clinics of North America* 7, no. 3 (1993): 631–45.

26. Eastern Breast Cancer Collaborative Group (EBCCG), "Systemic Treatment of Early Breast Cancer by Hormonal, Cytotoxic, or Immune Therapy," *Lancet* 339 (1992): 71–85.

27. Myers and Williams, "Role of High Dose Chemotherapy." Metastatic patients are commonly treated with hormonal therapy, such as tamoxifen. Approximately two-thirds of patients who fail hormonal therapy respond to cytotoxic therapy, although only one in five will achieve a "complete response." Complete response is defined as the disappearance of all measurable or assessable tumors for at least thirty days (ECRI, "High-Dose Chemotherapy"). Overall, the medical response duration is less than one year (Myers and Williams, "Role of High-Dose Chemotherapy").

28. Stephanie F. Williams, "Application of Peripheral Blood Progenitors to Dose-Intensive Therapy of Breast Cancer," *Breast Cancer Research and Treatment* 26 (1993): S25–9.

29. Initial developments in bone marrow and blood stem cell transplantation were related to concerns about the potential consequences of irradiation to humans following World War II. By the 1950s, initial animal studies indicated that viable cells from the spleen and marrow could circulate in the bloodstream and repopulate marrow ablated by irradiation (radioprotection) (Kenneth F. Mangan, "Peripheral Blood Stem Cell Transplantation: From Laboratory to Clinic," *Seminars in Oncology* 22, no. 3 [1995]: 202–9).

30. Garrett A. Smith and I. Craig Henderson, "High-Dose Chemotherapy (HDC) with Autologous Bone Marrow Transplantation (ABMT) for the Treatment of Breast

Cancer: No, the Jury Is Still Out," in *Important Advances in Oncology 1995,* Vincent T. DeVita et al., eds. (Philadelphia: J. B. Lippencott Company, 1995).

31. ECRI, "High-Dose Chemotherapy."

32. National Cancer Institute, *Research Report: Bone Marrow Transplantation and Peripheral Stem Cell Transplantation*, NIH Publication Number 95-1178 (1994).

33. ECRI, "High-Dose Chemotherapy."

34. A. Gratwohl and J. Hermans, "Bone Marrow Transplantation Activity in Europe 1992: Report from the European Group for Bone Marrow Transplantation," *Bone Marrow Transplant* 13, no. 1 (1994): 5–10.

35. ECRI, "High-Dose Chemotherapy."

36. F. R. Dunphy, G. Spitzer, A. U. Buzdar, et al., "Treatment of Estrogen Receptor-Negative or Hormonally Refractory Breast Cancer with Double High-Dose Chemotherapy Intensification and Bone Marrow Support," *Journal of Clinical Oncology* 8 (1990): 1207–16.

37. William P. Vaughan, "Autologous Bone Marrow Transplantation in the Treatment of Breast Cancer: Clinical and Technologic Strategies," *Seminars in Oncology* 20, no. 5, Suppl. 6 (October 1993): 55–8.

38. ECRI, "High-Dose Chemotherapy."

39. Three Phase III clinical trials supported by the National Cancer Institute have been under way and accruing patients for several years, as of this writing. Two of the studies are accruing women with Stage II or IIIA breast cancer, and the third is accruing women with Stage IV (metastatic or recurrent) breast cancer.

40. ECRI, "High-Dose Chemotherapy."

41. ECRI, "High-Dose Chemotherapy."

42. Physical and emotional frailty were a significant barrier or constraint to interviewing many women for this paper.

43. Aliza Kolker, "Thrown Overboard: The Human Costs of Health Care Rationing," in *Ethnographic Alternatives,* Carolyn Ellis and Arthur Bochner, eds. (Walnut Creek, Calif: Altamira, Press, forthcoming).

44. Robert N. Proctor, *Cancer Wars: How Politics Shapes What We Know and Don't Know about Cancer* (New York: Basic Books, 1995).

45. ECRI, "High-Dose Chemotherapy."

46. Gina Kolata, "Women Rejecting Trials for Testing a Cancer Therapy," *New York Times* (February 15, 1995): B1, B7.

47. K. Antman, J. P. Eder, A. Elias, et al., "High-Dose Combination Alkylating Agent Preparative Regimen with Autologous Bone Marrow Support: The Dana-Farber Cancer Institute/Beth Israel Hospital Experience," *Cancer Treatment Report* 71 (1987): 119–25; J. P. Eder, K. Antman, and A. Elias, "Cyclophosphamide and Thiotepa with Autologous Bone Marrow Transplantation in Patients with Solid Tumors," *Journal of the National Cancer Institute* 80 (1988): 1221–6; W. P. Peters, J. P. Eder, W. D. Henner, et al., "High-Dose Combination Alkylating Agents with Autologous Bone Marrow Support: A Phase I Trial," *Journal of Clinical Oncology* 4 (1986): 6446–54; R. B. Slease, J. B. Benear, G. B. Selby, et al., "High-Dose Combination Alkylating

Agent Therapy with Autologous Bone Marrow Rescue for Refractory Solid Tumors," *Journal of Clinical Oncology* 6 (1988): 1314–20.

48. Myers and Williams, "Role of High-Dose Chemotherapy."

49. K. Antman, L. Ayash, A. Elias, et al., "A Phase II Study of High Dose Cyclophosphamide, Thiotepa, and Carboplatin with Autologous Marrow Support in Women with Measurable Advanced Breast Cancer Responding to Standard-Dose Therapy," *Journal of Clinical Oncology* 10 (1992): 102–10; David M. Eddy, "High Dose Chemotherapy with Autologous Bone Marrow Transplantation for the Treatment of Metastatic Breast Cancer," *Journal of Clinical Oncology* 10 (April 1992): 657–70; K. F. Mangan, T. R. Klumpp, L. D. Glenn, and J. S. Macdonald, "High Dose Busulfan-Cyclophosphamide with Autologous Bone Marrow or Blood Stem Cell Rescue for Chemosensitive Stage IV Breast Cancer," *Journal of Cellular Biochemistry Supplement* 16, Part A (1992): 217; Myers and Williams, "Role of High-Dose Chemotherapy."

50. Eddy, "High Dose Chemotherapy."

51. J. O. Armitage, "New Frontiers in Cancer Chemotherapy?" *Journal of Clinical Oncology* 4 (1986): 1577–8.

52. W. P. Peters, M. Ross, J. J. Vredenburgh, et al., "High-Dose Chemotherapy and Autologous Bone Marrow Support as Consolidation after Standard-Dose Adjuvant Therapy for High-Risk Primary Breast Cancer," *Journal of Clinical Oncology* 11 (1993): 1132–43.

53. Lois J. Ayash, "High Dose Chemotherapy with Autologous Stem Cell Support for the Treatment of Metastatic Breast Cancer," *Cancer* 74 (1994): 532–5.

54. Thomas J. Smith, "Which Hat Do I Wear? (Physician Counsels Patient with Recurrent Breast Cancer Regarding Autologous Bone Marrow Transplantation)," *Journal of the American Medical Association* 270, no. 14 (1993): 1657–60.

55. Deborah R. Gordon, "Tenacious Assumptions in Western Medicine," in Lock and Gordon, *Biomedicine Examined*, pp. 19–56.

56. Gordon, "Tenacious Assumptions"; Gordon (p. 21) quotes Charles Taylor: "behind and supporting the impetus to naturalism . . . stands an attachment to a certain picture of the agent [actor]. . . . It shows us capable of achieving a kind of disengagement from our world by objectifying it. We objectify our situation to the extent that we can overcome a sense of it as what determines for us our paradigm purposes and ends, and can come to see it and function in it as a neutral environment, within which we can effect the purposes which we determine out of ourselves."

57. An advertisement commemorating the seventy-fifth anniversary of the American Cancer Society and appearing in a current journal for oncology specialists visually and verbally captures the progressive ideology. Above a picture of the entertainer Leslie Uggams, smiling ecstatically and clapping her hands, appear the lines, "There are three million Americans alive today who have had cancer. And now one out of two cancer patients get well!"

58. David N. Moolton, "Peripheral Blood Stem Cell Transplant: Future Directions," *Seminars in Oncology* 22, no. 3 (1995): 271–90.

59. Smith and Henderson, "High-Dose Chemotherapy (HDC)," p. 9.

60. Gordon, "Tenacious Assumptions," p. 21.

61. See, for example, the accounts of patients struggling to obtain HDC/ASCR treatments in Christina Middlebrook, *Seeing the Crab: A Memoir of Dying* (New York: Harper Collins, 1996); Aliza Kolker, "Thrown Overboard: The Human Costs of Health Care Rationing," in *Ethnographic Alternatives,* Carolyn Ellis and Arthur Bocher, eds. (Walnut Creek, Calif.: Altamira Press, forthcoming).

62. David Armstrong, "Clinical Sense and Clinical Science," *Social Science and Medicine* 11 (1977): 599–601.

63. This term refers to variation across different specialty groups within the medical profession.

64. Anselm Strauss et al., *Psychiatric Ideologies and Institutions* (New York: Free Press of Glencoe, 1964); Kathryn M. Taylor, "Physicians and the Disclosure of Information," in Lock and Gordon, *Biomedicine Examined*, 441–63.

65. Taylor, "Disclosure of Information," p. 444.

66. Another recent use of BMT is in the treatment of sickle-cell disease. Mark C. Walters et al., "Bone Marrow Transplantation for Sickle Cell Disease," *New England Journal of Medicine* 335 (1996): 369–76.

67. Strauss et al., *Psychiatric Ideologies*; Taylor, "Disclosure of Information."

68. NCI supports a large network of Community Clinical Oncology Programs (CCOPs), Cooperative Groups, and Cancer Centers that provide treatments and perform clinical trials. In 1994, NCI supported twenty-eight such centers along with thirty other centers receiving grant support. The CCOPs were established in 1983 as a network of community cancer specialists, primary-care physicians, and other health care professionals to conduct research on clinical treatment, prevention, and screening. The Clinical Cooperative Groups program conducts approximately thirty-five breast cancer treatment trials that enroll approximately 5,000 new patients each year. The comprehensive cancer centers are mandated to develop strong links with community physicians and support groups and to serve as a conduit for bringing treatment, prevention, and screening innovations into communities (Bruce Cheson, *Congressional Testimony before the Subcommittee on Compensation and Employee Benefits, Committee on Post Office and Civil Service: Autologous Bone Marrow Transplantation as a Treatment for Breast Cancer,* Federal Document Clearing House, August 11, 1994).

69. Kolata ("Women Rejecting Trials," p. B7) provides the following scenario: Among hospitals offering transplants is Hackensack Medical Center in New Jersey. Dr. Andrew Pecora, director of the bone marrow transplant program, said he gives women a choice of joining the national clinical trial or going ahead with a transplant independently. Of the sixty women who have had transplants at Hackensack in the last few years, only a few have joined the trial. "I have doctors call me up and say, 'Don't you dare offer my patient the clinical trial,'" Dr. Pecora said. He said some doctors give their patients chemotherapy before sending them to Hackensack, knowing it makes them ineligible for the trial.

70. Smith and Henderson, "High-Dose Chemotherapy (HDC)"; Eddy, "High Dose Chemotherapy"; Hillner, Smith, and Desch, "Efficacy and Cost-Effectiveness"; Vaughan, "Autologous Bone Marrow Transplantation"; Myers and Williams, "Role of High-Dose Chemotherapy."

71. W. E. Leary, "Payment Policy on New Treatments Draws Fire," *New York Times* (March 2, 1989): B14; L. E. Mortenson, "Tight-Money Casualties in the War on Cancer: Insurers Target Chemotherapy Payments," *Wall Street Journal* (May 11, 1989): A14; "The Price of Living," *NBC Dateline* (April 20, 1993).

72. K. Antman, L. E. Schnipper, and E. Frei, III, "The Crisis in Clinical Cancer Research: Third-Party Insurance and Investigational Therapy," *New England Journal of Medicine* 319 (1988): 46–8; G. P. Canellos, "Who Should Pay for Clinical Research?" *Journal of Clinical Oncology* 8 (1989): 1775–6; M. McCabe and M. A. Friedman, "Impact of Third-Party Reimbursement on Cancer Clinical Investigation: A Consensus Statement Coordinated by the National Cancer Institute," *Journal of the National Cancer Institute* 81 (1989): 1585-6; T. R. Spitzer, S. M. Swain, M. E. Lippman, and H. J. Deeg, "Reimbursement for Solid Tumor Autologous Bone Marrow Transplantation Trials: A Strategy for Ensuring Continuation of a Promising Therapy," *Cancer Investigation* 9 (1991): 93–7.

73. The *Bone Marrow Transplant Newsletter* is a resource available to patients and their families on-line through NYSERNet, Inc. We accessed the newsletter through the Community Breast Health Group, a community support and information group for breast cancer patients in Palo Alto, California. In addition to providing detailed scientific, financial, and legal information for patients considering a bone marrow transplant, the newsletter publishes an on-line discussion group for patients and families. Although oriented toward individual decision making, the materials published generally reflect a protransplant bias.

74. William P. Peters and Mark G. Rogers, "Variation in Approval by Insurance Companies of Coverage for Autologous Bone Marrow Transplantation for Breast Cancer," *New England Journal of Medicine* 330 (1994): 473–7.

75. Smith and Henderson, "High-Dose Chemotherapy (HDC)."

76. Peters and Rogers, "Variations in Insurance."

77. Anna C. Mastroianni, Ruth Faden, and Daniel Federman, eds., *Women and Health Research: Ethical and Legal Issues of Including Women in Clinical Studies* (Washington, D.C.: National Academy Press, 1994).

78. Robert J. Levine, "The Impact of HIV Infection on Society's Perception of Clinical Trials," *Kennedy Institute of Ethics Journal* 4, no. 2 (1994): 93–8; Levi, "Unproven AIDS Therapies."

79. The published report of a recent randomized controlled trial of HDC/ASCR justified the use of a particular chemotherapy agent. "While it may be argued that vincristine has marginal effects in breast cancer, the conventional-dose CNV regimen containing this drug was one with which this unit was familiar, and using a well-tested regimen for one of the treatment arms gave the opportunity to evaluate whether the response and response duration in this patient population conformed to previous experience" (W.R. Bezwoda, L. Seymour, and R. D. Dansey, "High-Dose Chemotherapy with Hematopoietic Rescue as Primary Treatment for Metastatic Breast Cancer: A Randomized Trial," *Journal of Clinical Oncology* 13 [1995]: 2488).

80. Kolata, "Women Rejecting Trials," p. B7.

Dick Willems

Outcomes, Guidelines, and Implementation in France, the Netherlands, and Great Britain

The relationship between outcomes data and what physicians do in everyday practice is far from straightforward. David Eddy has pointed to one of the sources of this problem: outcomes data are rarely generated within the patient population that physicians treat. They originate mostly from a highly artificial situation: controlled clinical trials or similar activities. Thus, family physicians treating eczema may not be helped by outcomes data generated within a tertiary-care hospital where only the more serious cases are seen.

A "device" is needed to connect outcomes data to the practical situation, and practice guidelines are such a device (there are many other names, such as "consensus recommendations," "protocols," or "standards," which I will not use here). So, one of the functions of practice guidelines is *translating* outcomes data into medical decisions. Just a few words on the term "translation" may be in order here.[1] Because of its double meaning, "translation" is a good term for describing what happens when scientific information or a technical innovation is transported to users. It involves not only rendering the same thing in a different language but also shifting and transforming and adapting it to the circumstances and desires of users. The acceptance of scientific insights or technical innovations thus involves their modification. This, I think, is what happens to outcomes data when they are translated into practice guidelines.

Guidelines have been developed, published, and disseminated in most Western countries during the last two decades, not only with the purpose of connecting data to practice but also for other goals: reduction of unjustified practice variations, improving the quality of care, allowing for medical audit, helping physicians negotiate with patients, and, finally (the most tricky one), cost reduction. The problem with the last goal is that practice guidelines sometimes do not make health care cheaper but more expensive (and, hopefully, better).[2]

This chapter has three parts: first, I will discuss the general outlines of the procedures for guideline development as they have been elaborated in France, Great Britain, and the Netherlands. Second, I will review some of the research on the implementation and acceptance of practice guidelines among physicians. The last part of the paper contains some reflections on the different purposes that guidelines are to serve and on the consequences for the extent of implementation that is both possible and desirable.

Development of Practice Guidelines

France

Although consensus conferences have been conducted in France since 1987 (generating some fifty consensus documents),[3] the systematic and nationwide development of practice guidelines is fairly recent in that country. After an unsuccessful attempt in 1987 (by INSERM),[4] a national program started at the end of 1993 in a rather stormy fashion. As a part of the two-yearly agreement on cost containment between physicians and insurance companies, the government demanded that obligatory guidelines (*références opposables*) be formulated in order to avoid unnecessary cost. Around twenty-five of these guidelines were elaborated in the last four months of 1993 by committees that were convened by the Caisses France. They concerned such issues as the number of ultrasounds administrated in normal pregnancy, the use of X rays to diagnose low back pain, etc. The content of the guidelines was more prohibitive than prescriptive. The most remarkable part of these documents, and the part that raised the most passionate reactions, was the sanctions paragraph: it was stipulated that those who, in the course of the year, generated frequencies above the guidelines would be subjected to a salary reduction equivalent to the extra cost they had generated.

The second phase of France's national guideline development program has consisted of a slower and more careful procedure (although guidelines are still developed at a staggering speed—thirty in one year!). Since 1994, the National Agency for the Development of Evaluation in Medicine (ANDEM) has prepared consensus documents that are used for educational purposes and the like; the Caisses Nationales and the Physicians' Syndicates take the most unambiguous from these recommendations as the basis for obligatory guidelines.

One of the distinctive elements of the recommendations developed by ANDEM is their *multidisciplinary* character. That is, they are prepared by both medical specialists and family physicians in mixed working groups. Moreover, a regional representation of the whole country is sought.[5]

Great Britain

In Great Britain, the King's Fund Centre organized national consensus procedures between 1984 and 1991. It was forced to stop these activities for two reasons: funding was becoming increasingly difficult, and the support for, and impact of, the statements were considered disappointing.[6] One of the interesting features of this program was the large involvement of the public in the conferences. Since 1991, there has been no systematic national guideline development program in Great Britain, although some professional organizations, such as the British Thoracic Society, have published national guidelines for well-defined conditions. On the other hand, there has been a tremendous amount of local guideline development. The most interesting feature of the British endeavor is precisely the local character and the emphasis put on "ownership" as a prerogative for implementation.

The Netherlands

In the Netherlands, instead of a multidisciplinary procedure, two parallel national procedures for guideline development exist. The first is restricted to family physicians, while the second addresses a general medical audience and mainly discusses problems in hospital medicine (although overlap between the two procedures exists). The hospital procedure, designed and operated by a specific bureau (CBO), is very similar to the consensus development program that exists in the United States. Since 1981, approximately fifty consensus documents have been produced.

The family physicians, represented by the Dutch College of General Practitioners, produce so-called standards for the ten thousand family doctors in Holland. The procedure they use is different from the second in various respects. First, the working groups preparing the guidelines consist exclusively of family physicians, and nonexperts are explicitly invited to participate. This fulfills a condition that British general practitioner Andrew Farmer has formulated thus: "Unless a guideline accurately reflects the routine working practices of most doctors it will act only as gold standard to be admired."[7] Second, guidelines, once they are finished, are sent to a random sample of fifty members of the college, who are invited to comment on issues (e.g. applicability in ordinary practice). These two characteristics of the procedure are part of the college's implementation strategy.

In the Netherlands, the somewhat surprising situation arises that generalists and specialists make distinct guidelines for the same condition. Thus, two slightly different guidelines exist for the treatment of asthma in children, one designed by the consensus organization and the other by the family physicians' college. In part, the family physicians have chosen to design their own guidelines for political reasons, that is, to guarantee their independence. There is also an epidemiological reason, however, that I alluded to in my introduction—that the difference in population should lead to different diagnostic and therapeutic strategies. In fact, this is another way of choosing a local strategy.

In the Netherlands the working groups preparing the guidelines take at least a year to discuss the available outcomes research, its relevance for family practice, and the translation of outcomes data into recommendations. This translation, in my view, is an activity in which hard data are mixed with softer data and with judgments about what is essential to family practice. Here is an example of such a translation: The working group on the guideline for the management of rheumatoid arthritis discussed the use of different tests for the disease. As with all tests, the predictive value of these tests depends on the population they are used in. These are quantifiable, hard outcomes data. The recommendation, however, that is given as to which test should be used under which conditions cannot be deduced from these data, because it involves discussions about, for instance, the acceptability of the risk of missing a diagnosis by not performing a test.

The fact that values play such a prominent role in guideline development raises two questions: first, *how* are values linked to outcomes data, and second, *who* should be involved in the process? For the answer to the first question, the working process of guideline-producing groups will have to be investigated, probably with ethnographic or similar approaches. The second question takes us to the politics of guideline development, and more specifically to the role of patients in it. In Denmark and Great Britain, the general public was invited to take part in guideline development in an attempt to make the process more democratic. This may seem to be an attractive option on the general level, but it will not solve the problem that arises when individuals do not agree with the guideline, even if it was produced "democratically." For this problem, the *flexibility* of guidelines seems a better option.

Recently two Dutch professors of general practice, in a criticism of what they take to be the implicit ideology of implementation studies—namely, that guidelines are there to be followed entirely and completely—proposed that the main role of guidelines is to function as agendas for policy making and audit in local groups of physicians.[8] They argued that strict adherence to guidelines is not to be sought and that deviations from them are always justified "because there are no normal patients." Guidelines, according to these two authors, should provide the basic material for the development of a critical attitude rather than a checklist to be used indiscriminately. Such a view, which is related to David Eddy's repartition of recommendations into standards, guidelines, and options,[9] could lead to a stratified system, in which some recommendations are so generally accepted as to become standards, whereas others are literally no more than guidelines and still others merely describe several options a physician or a patient can choose from.[10] To some extent, developments in France fit this idea: the largest part of the recommendations developed by ANDEM are guidelines and options, while only a minority are rewritten to become *références opposables*, obligatory standards.

The relationship between individual judgment and more or less universal guidelines is discussed explicitly in an editorial in the *British Medical Journal*: "Sooner or later the great debate between individual judgment and agreed standards will have to be held." This editorial locates much of the implementation difficulty in what it takes to be an understandable resistance of physicians: their fear of losing an essential part of their job, making clinical judgments. In other words, physicians fear the growth of "cookbook medicine."[11] The resistance of physicians against guidelines, however, in my view, is not so much concerned with clinical freedom (most often a suspect notion used by those who try to avoid accounting for what they are doing), but interference with what it means to be a physician. Stanley Reiser has defined the task of technology assessment as the investigation of the change in views about disease and about what medicine means by technological innovations.[12] I think the same applies to guidelines as an innovation in medicine. Many physicians realize that following a guideline may take an entire consultation and thus may distract physician and patient from elements that go beyond it but may be just as important, for instance, the meaning of complaints in the life history of a patient or within the context of his family. Instead of seeing guidelines and standards as a threat to the physician's independence or autonomy, I would say that they may restrict the physician's registers.

Implementation Strategies

In Europe there seems to be little opposition to the idea that medical practice can be regulated, to some extent, by guidelines. Physicians, policy makers, health insurers, and patients seem to accept that general protocols can be used to solve problems in individual health care. Especially physicians seem favorable to guidelines, provided they are developed by the profession and not by policy makers or third-party payers. But even if there is no great opposition to the principle of "guidelining" medical practice, guidelines are not followed by virtue of their mere existence. Instead they need to be actively implemented.

As has been suggested, two strategies for the implementation of guidelines in France exist: a "tough" one and a "soft" one. The tough strategy consists

158   Part II: Outcomes Data

of a system of sanctions that are applied to physicians who do not comply with the standards that are derived from the guidelines. The soft one is the publication of the existing guidelines; in 1994, two volumes were published containing twenty-eight practice guidelines. The organization of this type of implementation strategy is just beginning in France. Little can be said, up to now, about the effectiveness of this strategy.

In the Netherlands, the situation is more crystallized, probably because the two national programs for guideline setting have existed for a longer time. The College of General Practitioners has formulated a strategy for implementation that consists of the following elements:

1. Guidelines are all published in the journal for general practice.
2. Together with the published article, the GPs receive a plasticized card with the guideline in catchwords. It can be kept in a loose-leaf system designed for frequent use, both in the office and on house calls.
3. In 1993, a book was published containing the first thirty guidelines in a uniform format to be used in residency training.
4. A very recent development is the translation of some of the guidelines into computer menus that guide physicians on the spot in their treatment of patients.[13]
5. For most of the fifty existing guidelines, educational packages have been developed, available for use in groups of five to ten family physicians and consisting of a variety of educational formats—videotapes, structured patient cases, etc.
6. The implementation of guidelines is constantly monitored through a large computer network that is connected to a number of family practices nationwide.

The second guideline-developing body in the Netherlands, CBO, has less extensive implementation programs. Its main strategy consists of the publication of consensus statements in the *Dutch Journal of Medicine*; moreover, consensus documents are also available separately.

One development that is usually considered a strong incentive—although not intentionally so—for practicing within guidelines is their use in court. Although doctors are taken to court less frequently in Europe than in the United States, there seems to be a growth in European malpractice suits, and practice recommendations are undoubtedly going to play a role here. This, however, is still largely the future: in 1992 a review of court rulings in the Netherlands revealed one instance of the use of "consensus" as an argument in a disciplinary procedure.[14] There is concern, however, in the Dutch medical press that through increasing juridical use of guidelines, their uncertainty and relativity may be lost from sight.

A last implementation strategy, which is more developed in the United States than in Europe, is that insurance companies use the guidelines as part of the procedure for contracting physicians. Again, this is still a piece of science fiction both in the Netherlands and Great Britain, but in both countries discussion of such arrangements is starting.[15]

There is an interesting difference in the strategies for implementation between France and Great Britain. In France, there is a national program of guideline development that works rather top-down, whereas the concern for local development or local adaptation of national guidelines is very strong in Britain. As Jonathan Lomas has said in an important review article, "The most successful behavior change strategies operate at a more local level, and with more careful targeting, than is feasible with a national or regional consensus exercise."[16]

The Outcomes of Guidelines

There is little research on the actual success of the national guideline program in France, and this is understandable from the relatively recent start of the program. In the Netherlands, family physicians have investigated the effects of their guidelines almost from the start of the program. Different outcomes measures have been taken as an indicator of the effects of guidelines: first, *knowledge* about the existence of the guideline; second, *reported conformity* to the guideline; third, *actual conformity* to the recommendations. As an example, I will briefly discuss one of the most recent studies concerning the guideline on the treatment of non-insulin-dependent diabetes mellitus by family physicians.[17] The first guideline the college developed gave recommendations for this disease, and it was one of the most widely acclaimed, both by family physicians and by specialists. A study of its implementation, conducted in 1992 among seventy-three family physicians, compared reported with actual behavior to find that seven tested statements from the guideline were reported to be followed by between 30 and 90 percent of the physicians, while from chart reviews the compliance proved to range from 3 to 65 percent. Actual compliance was systematically lower than reported compliance by about 30 percent.

The question of whether patients get any better from guidelines has scarcely been addressed, but recently one such study has been done in Great Britain in a remarkably well-designed and extensive way.[18] In this experimental study, groups of ten GPs were invited to set standards for one of five common diseases in childhood (acute cough, acute vomiting, bed-wetting, itchy rash, and wheezy chest); for one of the other conditions the same doctors received a guideline that had been developed either by specialists or by one of the other groups of family physicians. For two diseases, other forms of medical audit were used, and for one disease, doctors did not receive guidance at all. Put very briefly, the result of the study of physician behavior was that the only significant change that could be found was related to guidelines developed by the groups themselves. In the British literature, there is consensus that some sense of ownership of the guideline is necessary to work with it.[19]

The second half of this British study was designed to measure the health outcome of the implementation of guidelines. Methodologically, this proved to be the most difficult part, since it is hard to pinpoint the exact contribution of the guideline to improvement (or deterioration) of the patient. Only one of the five tested guidelines seemed to result in significant improvement: patients with recurrent wheezy chest improved, both in medication compliance and in number of days of breathlessness. A problem in implementation of guidelines that is rarely pointed to is the sheer number of them. Especially family physicians and specialists with broad expertise, such as internists, have to know and cope with a staggering number of guidelines of a varying but sometimes rather demanding nature. The Dutch GPs have about fifty standards by now, and only very few of those necessitate less than minor adaptations in their daily practice. A recent editorial in the *British Medical Journal* says that "it is arguable whether any more guidelines should be drawn up until some of the barriers to implementation have been surmounted."[20]

It could be fruitful to view the extent to which physicians follow guidelines as similar to patient compliance. Just as physicians are concerned with the extent to which patients follow their advice, guideline developers are interested in the extent to which physicians comply with advice. Research on patient compliance has located resistance to advice in various areas, such as feasibility and consonance with the views patients and others in their environment hold about disease. One of the strategies that is advocated to improve patient compliance is to increase the patient's involvement in his own treatment program by delegating parts of the management to him; in other words, by creating ownership of the treatment. Physicians all know that obtaining compliance from patients is extremely hard, especially if it concerns long-term compliance, yet many guideline designers seem to expect that the compliance of physicians is much easier to obtain.

Guidelines change medical practice not only in the sense of turning it into an evidence-based activity. Their impact could well be more significant; they may change the nature of clinical practice and the nature of conversations and negotiations between physicians and patients. The political or ethical point about the kind of practice that is constructed along with these guidelines is rarely, if ever, addressed. Here, the help of theories from the sociology of innovations would be welcome. This type of investigation asks to what extent technological innovations, whether machines or procedures, incorporates a new definition of users (both physicians and patients). That, I think, is a basic question that is hardly talked about with regard to guidelines, and that has obvious ramifications in the implementation problem. For instance, guidelines and standards as they have been developed in the Netherlands are either disease-oriented or procedure-oriented. The number of complaint- or problem-oriented guidelines is low. It is probable that this will have an important impact on the way physicians work now: focusing on disease or on symptoms and their meaning for a patient. It is my view that implementation research should address such issues.

Conclusion: What Should Guidelines Do?

The effort of guideline construction, as it has been discussed in this chapter, is in itself a clear indication that outcomes data do not guide clinical practice on their own. The link between data and practice is to be *constructed* for two reasons. First, outcomes data always cover only a part of a medical consultation or procedure. For most of what physicians and patients do and say, there are no reliable data on outcomes. Second, outcomes data are always chance statements; they give the odds of success versus failure of a treatment or a diagnostic procedure. They state the chance that a treatment will lead to disappearance or alleviation of symptoms, or the chance that a diagnostic test will give information about the etiology of symptoms. The translation of such statements into medical action demands, first, a judgment about the desirability of the result and, second, a trade-off of chances. For instance, if patients with obstructive lung disease hear that lifelong inhalation of steroids would lower the chance of loss of mobility because of lung function decrease by, say, 60 percent, the question is whether they would consider continuous inhalations a worthwhile "investment." Some will and some will not.

In the case of the individual patient, this may be a difficult but not impossible decision. Practice guidelines try to do more: they advise about such decisions in all similar cases. Thus, guidelines on chronic obstructive pulmonary disease specify that patients with a certain severity of the disease should be advised to take lifelong steroid inhalations. That is, practice guidelines developed by a group of physicians try to specify diagnostic and treatment decisions that can only be made in conversations and negotiations with patients.

Guidelines are no more or less than one element in a decision-making process among others, and they may be (and often should be) overruled by other considerations, such as the relative importance of health as a goal for a patient. Implementation of guidelines, therefore, cannot mean anything else than that they obtain the role of a decision element. Not "following" guidelines but "using" them can be the only aim.

To my view, the concept of detailed guidelines, formulated at a national (or even global) level, is both sociologically and ethically problematic. Sociologically, because there is hardly any doubt that effective implementation of such guidelines is extremely difficult; and ethically, because it may, indeed, lead to the type of physician who stops thinking for herself. Ideally, the basic unit for practice improvement is the small group of local physicians, working either in a hospital or as family physicians. This does not mean that national consensus is useless, and not even that national organizations should refrain from giving detailed guidelines. It does mean that national consensus can only be obtained in very limited areas, where there is little discussion, and that guidelines should above all function as guidance for the discussion among physicians.

Nevertheless, practice guidelines are here to stay. Guideline developers are just beginning to see that designing them is the simplest part of the job. There is a growing awareness that ideals concerning implementation should be modest, as modest as with the long-term treatment of people with a chronic disease. Practice guidelines, especially those addressing clinical problems instead of single diagnostic and therapeutic procedures, can at most pretend to become elements within the negotiations between physicians and patients. Implementation of guidelines, then, should mean the degree to which they play a role in treatment, not the extent to which they are followed.

NOTES

1. This use of the term "translation" is developed in the work of the French sociologists Latour and Callon in the field of science and technology studies. They have shown that the spreading of innovations means their translation both in the linguistic sense of changing languages and in the physical sense of shifting. See, for instance, M. Callon, "Some Elements of a Sociology of Translation," in *Power, Action, and Belief: A New Sociology of Knowledge?* ed. John Law (London: Routledge, 1986), pp. 196–234.

2. A. McColl, "Implementing Clinical Guidelines: Guidelines May Not Be Cost Effective," letter, *British Medical Journal* 307, no. 6905 (1993): 678–9.

3. P. Durieux, "Les sociétés scientifiques soivent-elles participer à l'élaboration de recommandations de pratiques cliniques?" *Revue des Maladies Respiratoires* 11, no. 3 (1994): 223–5.

4. B. Stocking, B. Jennett, J. Spiby, *Criteria for Change: The History and Impact of Consensus Development Conferences in the UK* (London: King's Fund Centre, 1991).

5. Agence Nationale pour le Développement de l'Evaluation en Médecine, *Elaborations des recommandations et références médicales,* 1995.

6. Stocking, Jennett, Spiby, *Criteria for Change,* p. 4.

7. A. Farmer, "Medical Practice Guidelines: Lessons from the United States," *British Medical Journal* 307, no. 6899 (1993): 313–7.

8. N. P. Van Duijn, B. Meyboom-De Jong, "Between Gold Standard and Golden Calf: The Function and Application of College Guidelines," *Huisarts en Wetenschap* 38, no. 1 (1995): 3–7.

9. David Eddy, "Designing a Practice Policy: Standards, Guidelines, and Options," *JAMA* 37 (1990): 566–8.

10. R. Grol, "Standard of Care or Standard Care? Guidelines in General Practice," *Scandinavian Journal of Primary Health Care* 11, Suppl. 1 (1993): 26–31.

11. M. H. Liang, "From America: Cookbook Medicine or Food for Thought— Practice Guidelines Development in the USA," *Annals of the Rheumatic Diseases* 1, no. 11 (1992): 1257–8.

12. Stanley Reiser, "Assessment and the Technologic Present," *International Journal for Technology Assessment in Health Care* 2 (1986): 7 12.

13. G. G. Baily et al., "Implementing Clinical Guidelines: Computers Allow Instant Access," letter, *British Medical Journal* 307, no. 6905 (1993): 679.

14. F. Van Wijmen, R. Grol, "Juridische aspecten van standaarden in de huisartsgeneeskunde." *Huisarts en Wetenschap* 35, no. 6 (1992): 235–9.

15. National Council of Public Health, *Report on Quality Requirements: Good Staff Membership,* 1990; B. G. Charlton, "Management of Science," *Lancet* 342, no. 8863 (1993): 99–100.

16. J. Lomas, "Words without Action? The Production, Dissemination, and Impact of Consensus Recommendations" *Annual Review of Public Health* 12 (1991): 41–65.

17. G. P. J. M. Konings, D. Wijkel, G. E. H. M. Rutten, "Do Physicians Succeed in Working According to the College Guideline on Non-Insulin Dependent Diabetes?" *Huisarts en Wetenschap* 38 no. 1 (1995): 10–14.

18. North of England Study of Standards and Performance in General Practice, "Medical Audit in General Practice. I: Effects on Doctor's Clinical Behaviour for Common Childhood Conditions," *British Medical Journal* 304 (1992): 1480–4; North of England Study of Standards and Performance in General Practice, "Medical Audit in General Practice. II: Effects on Health of Patients with Common Childhood Conditions," *British Medical Journal* 304 (1992): 1484–8.

19. M. R. Partridge, "The Impact of Asthma Guidelines on Clinical Practice," *Monaldi Archives for Chest Disease* 48, no. 4 (1993): 367–8.

20. T. Delamothe, "Wanted: Guidelines That Doctors Will Follow," editorial, *British Medical Journal* 307, no. 898 (1993): 218.

*PART III: Ethical Considerations:
The Resolvable and the Intractable*

FRED GIFFORD
Outcomes Research and Practice Guidelines: Upstream Issues and Epistemological Issues

ROBERT M. VEATCH
Technology Assessment: Inevitably a Value Judgment

JAMES LINDEMANN NELSON
Clinical Judgment versus Outcomes Research?

SANDRA J. TANEBAUM
Say the Right Thing: Communication and Physician Accountability in the Era of Medical Outcomes

Fred Gifford

Outcomes Research and Practice Guidelines: Upstream Issues and Epistemological Issues

In response to concerns about cost containment and the quality of health care and to the belief that variation in medical practice may be due in significant part to uncertainty, there has been a great deal of effort to generate large volumes of outcomes data and produce practice guidelines on their basis.

"Outcomes research," or that part of it called "effectiveness research," carried out to discern "what works," involves examining large amounts of data about rates of various outcomes given various treatments. It typically involves statistical analyses of outcomes data drawn from very large databases (such as hospital and insurance records). Consensus panels and input from experts complement such information. "Practice guidelines" are generated on the basis of these data and expert opinions and serve as recommendations for practice.

There have been criticisms of both the outcomes research and practice guideline movement and of particular studies or recommendations, and there is perceived to be a resistance to, or at least a lack of adherence to, the recommendations. Claims that physicians often ignore or override practice guidelines or data arising from outcomes studies raise the following questions: If there is such resistance, why? In particular, do clinicians have good reasons for discounting outcomes data and practice guidelines? How should we respond to this nonadherence? Can we make clinicians more accepting of these guidelines, either by responding to their concerns with counterarguments or by addressing "upstream issues" by modifying the way the practice guidelines or outcomes assessments are generated? Or is the practice guideline project simply misguided and doomed to failure?

A useful place to begin the discussion is this: One can imagine a number of self-interested reasons (or motives) why physicians might criticize or decline to follow practice recommendations. For instance, guidelines may be seen as a threat to clinicians' professional autonomy and thus resisted, whether in an

168   Part III: Ethical Considerations

unreflective way or in a planned strategy to fight the movement. Yet clinicians may also sometimes have good epistemological or methodological reasons for being critical or dismissive of guidelines, such as legitimate criticisms of the way the knowledge is generated.

This tension exists even within one of the common responses made by clinicians, namely, that they want (or feel they ought) to use clinical judgment instead. But what is clinical judgment? Some describe it as a special skill clinicians have that is effective in solving problems and yet not reducible to rules or statistical reasoning. Others describe it as what clinicians say they are doing when they aren't able to do much more than guess. Since in the first case presumably we would say that clinical judgment should be respected and in the latter case not, it is particularly important that we be able to evaluate clinicians' reasons for not adhering to practice guidelines.

To address these questions, it will help to explore certain general issues concerning how data and guidelines can be open to challenge on grounds of being biased or value-laden and, more generally, what legitimate reasons one can have for not relying on them. This should help us to evaluate the decision not to follow a guideline or the results of a study and determine when it makes sense to press for adherence.

Outcomes Data versus Practice Guidelines: Descriptive versus Normative

One of the central distinctions to keep in mind is that between factual claims and normative claims. It is natural to view the project as the generation of guidelines about proper treatments based on careful and systematic examination of the data, and it may be tempting to see the whole process as a straightforward—if complicated—scientific exercise that will be adequately carried out as long as we enlist the best experts, are as careful as possible about scientific methodology, and gather as much data as possible. But this is a misleading picture.

It is one thing to make a statement of fact about the way the world is, another to make normative recommendations concerning what one ought to do. Thus there is a crucial difference between outcomes data and recommendations, such as practice guidelines. The former involve factual or descriptive claims, while the latter make normative or prescriptive claims. Moreover, in inferring a normative claim from any amount of outcomes data, one is implicitly bringing in some normative assumption, for example, about the appropriateness of the goal. And of course the possibility of different goals here is not trivial. Different patients may have different attitudes concerning the importance of attaining certain health goals and avoiding certain side effects. And there can be a tension between what is best for the individual patient and what is best for society (as, for instance, when cost containment is an issue).

This is often hidden in these discussions by saying that we are looking to find "what works"; but we must not be confused by this. To pick some outcome and say that if a method brings this about, then it "works" is to smuggle in a certain premise about values. Whether a procedure is appropriate or ought to be recommended cannot be determined simply by empirical inquiry.

All this might suggest that the main misgivings practitioners have would be with the practice guidelines, not the outcomes assessment—with a set of recommendations, not with statements about facts. Now, it is true that there are more ways to have (reasonable) objections to practice guidelines (recommendations) than to factual claims. But there are times when one can challenge "the facts." And in any case, sometimes the normative premise simply is not controversial whereas the factual claim that the treatment really would have a certain effect is. So we will be looking at both of these.

Explicit Reasoning versus Clinical Judgment

What is clinical judgment? How reliable (and hence valuable) is it? Does it conflict with (is it threatened by) an emphasis on outcomes data and guidelines? Statistical outcomes data would appear to be objective (in the sense of being less subject to bias than clinical judgment) and so more likely to be right. Further, such data and such methods of decision making, being more explicit and hence potentially public, better promote accountability for the clinical decisions made and enhance the opportunity for learning more about the decision process.

On the other hand, some worry about an uncritical reliance on objective data and explicit decision procedures.[1] The claim is that this yields too narrow a view of how clinical reasoning works when it works best and, further, that because the idea of relying only on the more objective data or guidelines is likely to be seductive, there will be a dangerous pull toward doing this, out of proportion to its true value. The claim is that there simply are no explicit rules for decision making, either for individual clinicians or for experts on consensus panels.

It is held that clinicians have a very valuable skill in coming to judgments in a way that cannot be specified by rules and that works not by considering the largest amount of statistical data possible and making calculations of probabilities but by looking carefully at the details of the individual case, analogizing to similar, familiar cases, and using intuition built up from years of clinical experience.

Yet when clinicians don't make judgments according to objective statistics, the question arises whether they are relying on sound reasons about a particular patient or on arbitrary factors, such as which procedures one happened to learn in medical school[2]—which are nonetheless experienced subjectively as clinical judgment. Those who favor statistical reasoning may suggest that differences of opinion or whatever we can't explain with a set of rational rules simply get labeled clinical judgment.

I believe that generating and encouraging the use of objective outcomes data is a worthy and realistic goal. But this must be done in a way that isn't too rigid, allowing some clinical judgment or discretion. Another worry is that a formal, statistical approach may not dovetail with the patterns of reasoning that clinicians in fact use, and so might not be the most efficient way to improve their behavior.[3] This general conclusion leaves us in a quandary: one needs to allow discretion, and yet one wants the "rules" to have some teeth in them.

A further point can be made. Insofar as we don't or can't say much specifically about how clinical judgment operates, there is the danger that it can be used as a sort of "smokescreen." One can always say that one has used one's clinical judgment. As a result, it is important to tease out more specific features of clinical judgment.

Briefly, clinical judgment is said to involve *intuitive* knowledge, *analogical* reasoning, *causal* (and temporal) reasoning about the disease process, and reasoning using *less quantitative* information. I will not take up these issues here, but only stress that examining these elements of clinical reasoning more carefully would enable us to say more about what counts as doing them well.

Perhaps we can say that when clinical judgment is allowed to trump practice guidelines, there should be an obligation to make the specific case for doing so and elaborate the virtues of the particular pattern of reasoning so as to respond to the charge that it is a smokescreen. It will in any case be difficult to resolve this debate between these different views of medical reasoning and knowledge.

Challenges to Objectivity

Granted, reliance on clinical judgment or less straightforward evidential considerations is at least problematic from the methodological and epistemic points of view. When there are objective data from outcomes assessment, it might be argued that these trump the considerations of clinical judgment. But in fact we need to think further about the objectivity or challengeability of the data that are contained in outcomes assessments and that inform practice

Outcomes Research and Practice Guidelines   171

guidelines, in order to clarify how strong or weak an argument clinical judgment would be up against.

Let us consider the concern that such data are open to bias or value-ladenness. Some of the ways in which information from outcomes data might be value-laden or otherwise challengeable may be obvious or surface cases. Just as a practitioner might refuse to follow practice guidelines because he knows he can make more money if he does not, a group of experts putting together a consensus document could be biased for similar reasons. But there will be deeper, more interesting cases of value-ladenness and subjectivity. Put another way, a given case might raise only practical issues (or involve rather straightforward biases or stubbornness), or it might raise deeper epistemological issues.

In surface cases, we may be able to correct for bias in straightforward ways. In deeper cases, it may be more difficult to strip away the bias, or to get rid of it by using better methods to generate the data or draw inferences from them. For instance, there may not be agreement about what method would be the right one. To get clearer about this, it will be useful to catalogue some of the ways a clinician might reasonably be skeptical that data or practice guidelines should be relied upon. It is helpful to conceptualize the situation in the following way: for it to be rational for you to carry out a certain action as a result of a certain body of evidence, you must have good reason to believe that the study provides an answer to "your" question.

For instance, your question may be about the relative efficacy of two drugs you are considering using. You may have determined that if the evidence shows that agent A is more effective than B in bringing about end point E, then you will treat using A. That evidence is the missing premise you look to the study to provide. From this perspective, we can distinguish different ways in which the evidence can fall short. It can be a matter of the study (in your judgment) either not answering any questions properly or answering some question, but not *your* question.

In the first case, you can take the study to have methodological flaws. For instance, you may believe the study was not being properly controlled or did not reach the proper level of statistical significance. As a result, you claim, the data really do not show what they are purported to show.

In the second case, you may be convinced that the study gives an answer to *some* question, but you don't take this to be *your* question. Rather than denying or being skeptical of the truth of the factual claim (the conclusion of the study), you deny that the claim is *relevant*. And there are various ways in which its relevance can be questioned. First, the data may concern a (somewhat) different causal context than the one you are interested in. It might be a matter of a different population, a somewhat different disease state, or differences in the treatment (such as dosage). A case of particular interest is "temporality": the treatment may have developed even over the time since the study, so that the earlier results are now of questionable value.

Second, the study may have defined "recovery" or "disease progression" in a way that you disagree with, or used death as the end point when this is not all you are interested in. Relatedly, we sometimes say that a study shows *statistical* significance but not *clinical* significance. The degree of effect found might be so small as not to make it worth changing the way you treat a certain condition.

There is a particular distinction that is especially important for our purposes: the difference between finding evidence of effectiveness and finding evidence of *cost*-effectiveness. There are, in effect, two different end points, one of most interest to the individual patient and the other of most interest to society (or the payer). Value judgments are, of course, involved here, controversial ones, and the idea that practice guidelines have been constructed with cost-effectiveness in mind can make a clinician resistant to following them.

Both kinds of challenges to a study's relevance raise the question whether we should view the results as *generalizable*, that is, transferable to some new causal context or end point. On the one hand, we presumably want to encourage practitioners to take these differences (between the various causal contexts and the various end points) into account (as part of critically evaluating studies) rather than blindly following recommendations. Hence, they certainly can count as legitimate reasons for overriding outcomes data or guidelines. On the other hand, there is a worry that any of these rationales could be "abused"—used as a rationale to cover up some other reason for not adhering to guidelines. That is, just as in the case of *general* reference to clinical judgment, it can be "too easy" to use one or another concern about the data's relevance as an excuse to ignore guidelines. After all, the context will *always* be different in some way or other.

Further Challenges to Relevance

I want to describe more fully three deeper, subtler ways in which data or guidelines may not be able to be completely objective or value-free. One concerns the setting of statistical-significance levels, another description, another ambiguity of end points. Each of these involves ambiguity about the question a study is to answer or about the criteria for what counts as an answer. Thus, each raises questions about whether we can generalize as well as whether we should seek an upstream solution to the problem of nonadherence to practice guidelines by collecting data or generating guidelines in a different manner.

Statistical-Significance Levels

There is a quite general way in which value judgments might be said to be infused into inferences or conclusions of scientific studies, but it applies with a special importance in the case of medical knowledge, based as it is on statistical data from studies of populations of individuals. The argument, advanced by Rudner, is this: No empirical claim is ever proved or completely confirmed.[4] Any amount of evidence will allow us to assert a given claim only with some degree of confidence less than certainty. Thus, the decision to accept a certain scientific claim as true (to adopt it into our corpus of knowledge) requires judging that this statement is well enough confirmed to warrant accepting it. In the case of judging statistical hypotheses, we often go along with a particular standard "confidence level," but in fact there is a judgment to be made concerning whether this is "the right" standard to use in a given case.

Reflection on the problem reveals that this decision depends on the seriousness of the consequences of making a mistake (accepting a false hypothesis or rejecting a true hypothesis). But this is a matter of judging the value or disvalue (seriousness) of the various possible outcomes. In the case of medical hypotheses, these possible outcomes of the decision to accept a claim as well enough confirmed or reject it as not well enough confirmed will include such actions as having some ineffective treatment become available or standard or keeping an effective therapy from being available. These can be seen to be a matter of moral value judgments, ones that different people may make differently.

So the decision to accept a medical claim requires the value judgment that the degree of confirmation is high enough. What follows? First, Rudner takes his argument to have quite general application. His goal is to argue that scientists in their role as scientists must make value judgments and hence cannot be value-neutral. While a variety of responses question whether this conclusion follows for all of science (especially "pure science," if we can separate such a thing out from more applied science),[5] it seems pretty clear that it does apply to medical knowledge of the sort at issue here.

Further, note that while it is simplest to see in the case of judging the statistical significance of a set of statistical data from a certain population, the argument should apply to all sorts of medical scientific claims, including various bits of background knowledge. The operative premise is that evidence comes in *degrees*, that (in the case of empirical claims) it never reaches *certainty*, and hence that we have to decide if it is *enough*.

It is not implausible, then, to suggest that such value-ladenness pervades much of medical knowledge. Relatedly, values don't simply come into play where things have gone wrong, where there is a bias that should have been corrected. Further, if the value judgments at issue are not universally shared, this would appear to be a basis for possible disagreement over the firmness of the supposedly established medical facts. Finally, given the nature of the problem, it does not appear that we can solve the problem by determining the "right" level of statistical confidence.

The Description of Variables

A second way in which we may see elements in scientific statements that can be challenged as nonobjective relates to the way variables are described. This is a general phenomenon that applies across science. Alan Fleischman has nicely illustrated ways in which the data concerning neonates may not be exactly what they seem to be and how there are values involved in the data itself.[6] Thus, for example, various data are cited correlating gestational age with some other feature, such as probability of survival (or a certain expected quality of life). The naive observer might assume that these are fairly "hard" data. But because there is known to be an uncertainty of seven to ten days in dating a pregnancy, these data are not as accurate a description of the real world as one might hope or believe. If one naively relied on these data, one would not be as successful as one would expect in avoiding certain types of errors.

One may conclude that data are often not as "hard" as they may seem. Or one might describe the "take-home lesson" thus: to know properly how to interpret the data, it is often important to have a good understanding of the process by which they are generated. The description itself may not tell the whole story and may be misleading. Of course, if you were to make sure that everyone knew this (and had it clearly in mind), writing it in next to each chart or table in the published study, then this might not be a problem. The problem occurs when someone doesn't know this and so views the data as meaning more (in terms of accuracy) than they in fact do.

Note that what this case involves is a random scatter of inaccuracy in the data. The problem is created not by differences in value judgments but simply by a failure to understand the level of accuracy of the results. Still, it could be said (à la Rudner) that the decision to put the information in a table without comment involves a judgment that the consequences of relying naively on the data won't be that serious. This is indeed a value judgment—a controversial one. For being seven to ten days off may lead to categorizing a fetus as viable when it is not or nonviable when it is.

It might be suggested that this problem be solved by having the creators of practice guidelines include everything—all uncompiled data points and all features of the data collection situation. For then no controversial judgments would have to be made, and no one would be misled. But of course it is not really possible to make things watertight; it is more reasonable to recommend to creators of guidelines that they be careful to keep in mind which claims or kinds of data are likely to be controversial.

Consider another example, also from Fleishman, in which a value component is more directly implicated in "hard data": gestational age is correlated with "intact survival," defined as having an IQ of 85 or above and not having cerebral palsy or a hearing or visual impairment. The obvious way to read the data so correlated is as an indication of whether there was a good outcome. It is clear that value judgments inform this particular way of linking one set of facts (gestational age) with another (IQ and presence or absence of certain impairments) through a value-laden term ("intact survival"). (The issue is intensified by the decision not to count death as a bad outcome or to view the survival of an abnormal child as a worse outcome.) If the user of the information does not realize this, incorrect inferences will be drawn.

This example, like the previous one, forces an examination of the process by which the data are "generated," but the concern is not that one cannot always be completely objective in assigning an individual to a given (perhaps objective) category. Rather, decisions have to be made about how to delimit categories in the first place. Thus, simply increasing the *accuracy* of category assignments won't solve the problem of the initial value-ladenness of category definitions.

There are, of course, many examples of this in the sciences. A common one concerns specifying the meaning of normality. Another example from behavioral studies is when animal and human behavior is described with terms such as "aggression" or "dominance." In all these cases, different people may define the term differently, explicitly or implicitly. How should we respond? Is this sort of "invisible" ambiguity of categories bad? Is it avoidable? Data in the gestational-age case might be said to be "compiled data," that is, organized in certain ways for certain analytic purposes. To present information in a chart or table, one must at the outset decide which are the relevant categories (and what their boundaries are). But it seems plausible that some data are more "raw"—a bunch of data points. Perhaps one could always go back and say exactly what one's observations were, and thus specify what the raw (that is, objective) data were.

Researchers typically don't do this. Could they? Could they make sure that they provide the raw data as well, or refrain from compiling data in charts? There is, first, a technical problem concerning regress: If you want data absolutely free of value or particular categories, then you really have to go a very long way back into the process of generating the data. Even when you get to what look like the bare observational statements that scientists would make in the course of the study, it is not clear that those data would be pristine. Observation statements are never entirely free of theory.

In response, it might be argued that it isn't necessary to make our observations pristine, but we can try our hardest to make our concepts as clean and neutral as possible. The "in principle" problem would remain, but it wouldn't have much practical impact. For example, it wouldn't count as any reason to be skeptical about generating a database and practice guidelines made on the basis of it.

But would it make sense in terms of communicating knowledge to try to locate it as far back as possible? It would probably not facilitate communication to provide so much complicated information. There is inevitably a tension between increased neutrality and the ease and effectiveness of communication. How best to deal with this isn't obvious, but the analysis does suggest that the solution isn't to try to create a perfect database that will preclude all conflict. Rather, one needs to be as careful as feasible and, when there is resistance, explore this as a possible explanation.

The Ambiguity of End Points or Goals

Finally, I want to elaborate on a particular problem concerning relevance and generalizability. There are two important points here. First, difficulty agreeing about the appropriateness of particular data and guidelines derives in significant part from a lack of agreement over choice of end points. Second, at a deeper level, it may be in part a result of uncertainty concerning whether different end points are at issue. I will illustrate this by considering successively more complicated cases.

Sometimes you (as a clinician, "downstream") may be presented with data (or summary information such as practice guidelines) that are clearly about a different end point or question from the one that immediately concerns you. For example, suppose you are given the results of a well-designed randomized controlled trial comparing survival rates from two different drugs but you are a nutritionist trying to decide between two different nutritional regimens. Quite simply, these data are not relevant to your question and thus will quite rightly not move you to take any action different from what you would have done without them.

At other times, the fact that data presented to you are about a different end point or question will be less clear. Suppose, for example, you are given the results of a well-designed trial comparing treatments that you would consider using; indeed, you had specifically in mind the question of which of these to use. But the study involved a different population from yours—patients who are sicker, or less ill, than yours.

You might be right to worry about the applicability of these data, but it's not as though it's irrelevant (or at least obviously irrelevant), as in the first case. Perhaps it would be possible to generalize from that context to yours. Whether and how to do this will be a controversial matter, for we don't know well enough when it is appropriate to extrapolate: we don't have enough studies or adequate background knowledge. In fact, there will be a continuum of cases between the studies and target populations from those different only in trivial ways to those different in very profound ways. There will be some cases where the differences are clear and some where they are not.

The last two cases I want to consider concern differences in end points rather than in causal background. More important, they involve different value judgments about what end points are important: clinical effectiveness versus cost-effectiveness.

Suppose you are given a guideline based on studies you respect suggesting that treatment A should be given over treatment B, where A is said to be more cost-effective. But what *you* want to know is which is more effective, regardless of cost. Like the previous scenario, this may also seem pretty straightforward, on the face of it not requiring a deep analysis of, for example, what the nature of the data is. Rather, the data aren't relevant to your goals—unless, of course, the cost differential is so large that the more cost-effective treatment becomes perforce the most effective one to offer your particular patient. The issue of whether physicians should take up the cause of cost containment or rationing is a deep question, but it's not one about the nature of the data. It's a deep *ethical* question rather than a deep *epistemological* question.

This isn't to say that there couldn't be epistemological questions at issue here as well, of course. There could be ambiguity in the minds of those who collected the data (or compiled them) as to whether the goal was effectiveness or cost-effectiveness. (Indeed, if the data are drawn from many sources, some data may have been collected in relation to effectiveness and other data in relation to cost-effectiveness.) Further, impressions (perhaps incorrect) by downstream physicians of the intent (and method of data collection) of those upstream can also be a source of difficulty, particularly where expert opinion is at issue.

Finally, consider a case where guidelines are based in part on clinical judgment of expert physicians judging intervention A to be preferable to intervention B. The downstream physician may wonder whether the experts were judging which intervention was most effective or most cost-effective. And it isn't simply that the intended goal was not published with the recommendation, for the experts might well have been asked, What would you *do?* (This would be the most realistic question.) But one cannot tell from just this which goal is involved, effectiveness or cost-effectiveness.

Even if they are in fact asked the specific question, What would be most cost-effective? there remains some ambiguity, for this may be different from the way the expert usually thinks the matter through. Since expertise involves tacit knowledge that cannot be reduced to explicit rules, perhaps we could not expect experts' judgments to be as reliable outside the question of what they would in fact do as practicing clinicians faced with the given treatment choice.

Given these sorts of reflection on how medical knowledge is generated and transmitted, how might we respond to physicians' resistance to practice guidelines based on outcomes research?

In more complicated cases of value-laden information, it is not clear we can always or easily strip away values, biases, and mistakes and make some pronouncement about what the objectively correct empirical claim or clinical decision is. The implications of this deserve to be thought through further, but we cannot simply dismiss clinicians when they argue against adhering to guidelines on the grounds that the guidelines are "value-laden" and not sufficiently objective.

It also seems that uncertainty about the goals of those involved in constructing particular guidelines can breed mistrust of the entire process by which they are developed and promulgated. It is one thing for those downstream to have a particular objection to one of the methods used in gathering and compiling information and generating guidelines; it is another for them to be uncertain about the process and "assume the worst."

We may never be able to overcome all of the concerns physicians raise against outcomes data and practice guidelines, but we should strive to remove unnecessary barriers. We should allay doubts as to what the data and guidelines are *about* and reassure clinicians about the reasoning that informs guidelines—who compiled the data (and recommendations) and by what methods—not only on grounds of honesty but for pragmatic reasons as well. Addressing such upstream issues can help foster downstream understanding.

NOTES

1. Sandra Tanenbaum, "Knowing and Acting in Medical Practice: The Epistemological Politics of Outcomes Research," *Journal of Health Politics, Policy, and Law* 19, no. 1 (1994): 27–44; "What Physicians Know," *NEJM* 329 (1993): 1268–71.

2. David Eddy, "Variations in Physician Practice: The Role of Uncertainty," *Health Affairs* 3 (1984): 74–89.

3. Tanenbaum, "Knowing and Acting in Medical Practice"; "What Physicians Know."

4. Richard Rudner, "The Scientist qua Scientist Makes Value Judgments," *Philosophy of Science* 20 (1953): 1–6.

5. Richard Jeffrey, "Valuation and Acceptance of Scientific Hypotheses," *Philosophy of Science* 23 (1956): 237–46; I. Levi, "Must the Scientist Make Value Judgments?" *Journal of Philosophy* 57, no. 11 (1960): 345–56.

6. Alan R. Fleischman, "Outcomes Data and Low Birth-Weight Babies," paper presented at a meeting of The Hastings Center project "Technology Assessment: Uses, Context, and Interpretation," 13 December 1993, Briarcliff Manor, N.Y.

Robert M. Veatch

Technology Assessment: Inevitably a Value Judgment

"Technology assessment" is a systematically ambiguous term. Its ambiguity causes serious problems for policy makers and clinicians. On the one hand, "assessment" sometimes refers to the scientific study of the potential *effects* of a medical intervention. As such, technology assessment is often thought in the ideal to be scientific, objective, and value-free. On the other hand, "assessment" sometimes refers to judgments about the benefits and harms anticipated from medical interventions and when they should be pursued. They attempt to tell when a treatment is "medically indicated," "appropriate," or a "treatment of choice." They attempt to tell how patients should be "managed."[1] In this second sense technology assessment necessarily involves value judgments. Even in the ideal case deciding that something is *beneficial* or *harmful*, deciding something is *indicated* or *ought* to be used in particular circumstances always has to involve judgments about values that in principle cannot be determined by science alone.[2] Words like "beneficial," "harmful," "indicated," and "ought" necessarily convey evaluations that go beyond the scope of what modern practitioners of science consider scientific.

Determining what the expected effect of an intervention will be can, in principle, never tell whether that effect is good or bad, to be preferred or not. It can never tell how the effect compares, in evaluative terms, with other options. Any assessment of technology assessment will have to provide an adequate understanding of the relation between knowing the effects of a treatment and knowing how valuable the treatment is. Without knowing the value of the treatment one can, in principle, never know whether the treatment is worth pursuing.

The Function of Technology Assessment: The Received Wisdom

The critical question for this project is, Is technology assessment supposed to provide facts without value judgment, or is it supposed to provide the necessary value framework for making medical decisions? The received wisdom among many doing and using technology assessments is that high-quality, objective, scientific assessment of a technology will provide the basis for making correct clinical and public-policy decisions. It is as if the generation of outcomes data, cost assessments, and other ideally objective findings based on impeccable scientific methodologies, such as randomized clinical trials, can lead directly to decisions about which treatments are appropriate in various medical circumstances.

"Technology assessment" is a general term covering a range of activities. Some terms, such as "outcomes research," imply that the objective is to find facts, in particular to determine what the outcomes will be from various interventions. If that were all there were to outcomes research, it would have the trappings of a scientific activity. It would provide data upon which clinicians, patients, and policy makers could impose a set of values to determine whether the expected is simply the indication that an intervention might produce a certain effect.

The Patient Outcomes Research Team (PORT) studies, funded by the Agency for Health Care Policy and Research (AHCPR), are good examples of the first use of "technology assessment"; these studies seek to establish the outcomes of treatment intervention, such as whether radical prostatectomy and radiation therapy have an effect on localized prostate cancer.[3] Other technology assessments make clear that their intention is to go well beyond fact finding. *Practice guidelines* or *treatment protocols* clearly imply that the goal of their creators is to direct a treatment course or at least guide it. For example, AHCPR has produced a series of fifteen *Clinical Practice Guidelines,* all of which provide not only detailed descriptions of effects of an intervention but also recommendations for treatment and values to be pursued in "managing" patients.

Still other technology assessments sit ambiguously between the goals of fact finding and prescription. National Institutes of Health (NIH) Consensus Development Conferences have as their stated purpose to "evaluate publicly scientific information concerning biomedical technology and arrive at a Consensus Statement that . . . will serve as a contribution to scientific thinking about the technology under consideration."[4] In fact, if one examines the questions posed by the organizers of these conferences, it is clear that they sometimes want the conferees to reach a definitive consensus on questions of fact. For example, the consensus conference on gallstones and laparoscopic cholecystectomy asked the apparently scientific question, "What are the results of laparoscopic cholecystectomy compared with open cholecystectomy and other available treatments?"[5] Other times they ask questions that require bold and blatant value judgments by the conferees. The same gallstone conference asked,

"Which patients with gallstones should be treated with laparoscopic cholecystectomy?"[6] This a question that required judgments about risks to first- and third-trimester fetuses, and patients with end-stage liver disease, as well as more usual value judgments about whether anesthesia and other risks are justified by the envisioned benefits, compared with the risks. The conference on dental sealants in the prevention of tooth decay asked apparently factual questions such as, "How effective are sealants?" and asked clearly normative questions such as, "What should be the research priorities for sealants and their implementation?" Some of the questions combined both factual and evaluative questions, such as, "What are the clinical procedures involved in successful sealant application, and what training and education are required?"[7]

This chapter argues that technology assessment necessarily involves value judgments, and this is most easily demonstrated in treatment guidelines and other technology assessment that lead to treatment recommendations. A recommendation is, by its very nature, a statement that contains some normative prescription—a value judgment. This claim is explained in the next section by outlining the logical structure of clinical decisions; the succeeding section examines treatment guidelines and protocols to demonstrate that they make value judgments and necessarily go beyond the science. Guidelines and protocols evaluate the science and use somebody's values to decide what *ought* to be done in light of the data. The final section examines outcomes research, PORT studies, Office of Technology Assessment (OTA) reports, and NIH consensus development conferences that focus mainly on fact finding. This chapter argues that even those who eschew value judgments necessarily incorporate normative and conceptual commitments that shape the data and inevitably frame the decisions that clinicians, patients, and policy makers reach.

The Theoretical Structure of Clinical Decisions

Any clinical decision can be reduced to a formal syllogism of the following form:

If conditions A,B,C,D,E exist, then one should do X.

Conditions A,B,C,D,E exist.

Therefore, one should do X.

All clinical decisions can be analyzed into this form (as can all publicpolicy and other decisions). The second premise, the minor premise, will always contain fact claims. The placeholders—A,B,C, etc.—symbolize medical-fact claims that come from diagnostic tests, pharmacological facts, and the findings reported in outcomes research, as well as fact claims from other areas, including law, economics, sociology, and psychology. The minor premise for a patient with pneumonia, for example, might include medical facts that lab tests are positive for pneumococcus bacillus, that penicillin has a high rate of overcoming pneumonia and minimal side effects, and that the patient reports no history of anaphylactic reaction to penicillin. The minor premise could also include facts from other disciplines, including the legal fact that penicillin is a legally available drug with Food and Drug Administration (FDA)–approved labeling, etc., and the economic fact that resources made available to obtain penicillin might exclude other interactions.

Even if one assumes that the conditions in the minor premise are knowable by medical science, clearly the major premise is not. The major premise of the clinical decision-making syllogism must always contain a normative judgment such as represented in "one ought to do X." If the conclusion contains a prescription—a recommendation or order for a drug, surgical procedure, or any other action—the major premise contains a value judgment. The "ought" judgment cannot come directly from the science. It must be imported from some system of beliefs and values. In clinical decisions the beliefs and values have historically been the clinician's. In postmodern medical ethics with a commitment to patient autonomy, it is increasingly claimed that it is the patient's system of beliefs and values that ought to supply value judgment in the major premise. In public-policy decisions, the values of the broader society might serve this function.

Practice Guidelines and Treatment Protocols

Practice guidelines, treatment protocols, and other technology assessment devices that purport to guide, direct, recommend, or instruct clinicians in making decisions necessarily provide all three elements of the clinical syllogism. They draw on outcomes research, consensus conferences, and more traditional clinical trials to provide the medical data that fit into the minor premise.

Practice guidelines and treatment protocols, by necessity, go beyond the medical facts supplied by the scientific disciplines related to medical research. Although the writers of the guidelines and protocols often do not realize the fact, they incorporate—by implication in the minor premise—purported facts from other disciplines. Consider, for example, whether protocols for metastatic cancer should include in the treatment options the possibility of physician-assisted suicide or euthanasia. Almost no protocols include that option, in part because it is correctly believed that such options are illegal. Likewise, heroin is not a treatment option for severe pain, not because it is necessarily ineffective but because it is correctly believed to be illegal in the United States. Sociological and psychological facts are also often incorporated into treatment protocols.

Even if the writers of the protocols and the clinicians that use them can claim real expertise on the medical facts, they normally have no such claims to expertise on facts in other disciplines. Thus, there is already some reason to be suspicious that groups that write protocols do not necessarily have the scientific skills necessary to support all the relevant facts for a clinical recommendation.

The more obvious implication of the clinical treatment syllogism is that even if the protocol and practice guideline writers can assume that they have all the relevant facts of the minor premise correctly assessed in a value-free and reliable manner, reasons exist to question the major premise. It does not automatically follow from the fact that the patient has a bacillary form of pneumonia and has no history of anaphylaxis that the patient *should* take penicillin. True, almost all people reach that conclusion, but if they do, it is because they share a set of values that appraises the potential effects of the penicillin, compares those to the effects of other treatment options, and concludes that the effects of the penicillin are, on balance, better. That conclusion is not merely scientific; it assesses medical and other facts, imposes a set of values on the evidence, and concludes that one ought to take the penicillin. The nonscientific, normative nature of these decisions becomes apparent if one considers that a Christian Scientist might fully accept all the relevant facts of the minor premise and still deny that one ought to take penicillin. What is more important, some patients who make no special religious assumptions may, under special circumstances, deny the moral and other normative content of the major premise.

A terminally ill ninety-year-old patient with metastatic cancer may question whether it is better to take penicillin and live than refuse it and die. Medical science alone can never establish definitively that it is right to take penicillin when one has pneumonia. While medical science can always identify the effects of an intervention, only a patient can decide on what effects to prefer, and each patient brings unique values to a treatment decision. These unique values cannot be reflected in clinical practice guidelines.[8]

All practice guidelines and treatment protocols that recommend how a patient should be treated under certain conditions supply not only the diagnostic, prognostic, and pharmacological facts but also the other relevant nonmedical facts and the religious, philosophical, or other normative values that lead to the judgments about how the patient should be treated. For example, the guideline *Management of Cataract in Adults* includes the statement that the goal is to "maintain and restore autonomy through appropriate treatment to remove the disability."[9] In the guideline *Management of Cancer Pain: Adults*, the writers make the recommendation that "the clinician's ethical duty—to benefit the patient by relieving pain—supports increasing doses [of opioids], even at the risk of side effects."[10] Surely, that is not a conclusion of medical science, no matter how plausible the ethical opinion is among many cultural groups. In some of the guidelines some evaluative judgments are more subtle but, nevertheless, clearly convey value choices. In the guideline *Depression in Primary Care: Detection, Diagnosis, and Treatment*, the authors transfer some of the value choices to the clinician, as when they say that "if panic disorder and major depression are both present and the panic disorder has been present without episodes of major depression in the past, the clinician must judge which is the most significant condition."[11] In the guideline *Managing Otitis Media with Effusion in Young Children*, one of the many ways in which the value judgment of the writers is manifest is in how they handle the problem of whether to recommend intervention when the evidence of effect is not definitive. In discussing adenoidectomy for uncomplicated middle-ear effusion in the child younger than age four when adenoid pathology is not present, they say that, "based on the lack of scientific evidence," the treatment is not appropriate.[12] On the previous page, however, when faced with a situation where they lack evidence, they reach the opposite conclusion, saying, "Although there is insufficient evidence to prove that there are long-term deleterious effects of otitis media with effusion, concern about the possibility of such effects led the panel to recommend surgery [bilateral myringotomy with tube insertion for the child who has had bilateral effusion for a total of three months and other conditions]."[13] These are just a few of the countless value judgments made in the practice guidelines. Every time a procedure is recommended, a value judgment is made that takes the authors beyond the science. It is not that the judgments are implausible; it is simply that they do not come from the data.

 The only plausible conclusion is that all attempts to formulate practice guidelines or treatment protocols necessarily import moral and other value judgments from religious, philosophical, and other systems of belief and value from outside medical science. This partially explains why some clinicians offer resistance to treatment protocols, even those formulated by AHCPR and other bodies capable of providing the highest-quality research in medical science. Undoubtedly some clinicians might deviate from the recommendations of protocols and guidelines even if they believed the data to be valid and had perfect knowledge of it, because they might still reject the normative structure placed on the data by writers of the protocols. If clinicians placed less value on the autonomy of the elderly and more value on the efficiency of those in the labor force, clinicians might reach different conclusions about cataracts.

186 Part III: Ethical Considerations

If clinicians had a strong commitment to preserving life regardless of the pain, clinicians might be less willing to risk side effects of opioids. It is not clear why the clinician's determination of whether panic disorder or depression is more "significant" should be the definitive value. Nor is it clear why the panel's willingness to intervene in the face of insufficient evidence in one case but not the other should be definitive. Even if clinicians know exactly the effect of an intervention, clinicians cannot directly conclude whether that effect is a good or a bad one or how the various value tradeoffs should be made.

In the case of otitis media, the guideline makes clear that there is a statistically significant improvement in clearance of effusion at one month, while there is no difference at two months and no evidence of prevention of long-term hearing loss. Clinicians facing a child with otitis media may place more emphasis on short-term effects than do researchers who can show that there are no measurable long-term effects from the infection. Even if the protocol writers have a perfect account of the effects of administration of an antibiotic, they always place value on those effects. If the protocol writers focus exclusively on long-term effects while the clinician worries about the short-term, reversible consequences as well, the clinician may disagree with the writers of the protocol without denying that the writers have the best available estimate of the medical facts.

Moreover, just as clinicians may bring different values to the data than the protocol writers, so patients and their families may evaluate the outcomes differently from their clinician. That has led ethicists to claim that in principle, no clinician can ever know what is the best treatment for a patient without finding out what value system should be used for deciding benefits and harms. If we assume that the patient's values should be dominant in clinical decisions, then the only way that the clinician can know what is the best treatment for the patient is to turn to the patient, that is, ask the patient to evaluate treatment options and pick the one that fits the patient's value system.[14]

In the case of a patient incapacitated to make health care decisions and who has never chosen and expressed a set of values (e.g., pediatric patients with otitis media), the choice of the proper value system is more complicated. Increasingly society recognizes that the parent or other familial surrogate should select the values, provided they are within reason.[15] Normally, public agencies—courts and child-protection agencies—determine whether the family must be overridden. In any case, there is no reason to assume that the clinician's values are the appropriate ones to impose on the medical data.

Likewise, the values of the protocol writers cannot be assumed to be the definitive ones for making treatment recommendations. Assuming that the treatment protocol–writing group has definitive expertise in deciding the relevant medical facts, they should not be presumed to be authoritative in deciding which values to use. For some public-policy purposes the proper values may not be those of the individual patient; they may be those of the society.

Some may argue that practice guidelines and treatment protocols are written by groups of experts and this neutralizes the biases of individual experts. Even if biases are lessened, there is no reason to assume that the experts in the group writing the protocol represent either the individual patient or the society at large. Even in the case of public policy, for example, treatment protocols for mandatory immunizations or public-health food screening, the average values of the group writing a protocol might match those broader values, but good reason exists to doubt that this is always true. Those who emerge as experts in a field such as medicine may have value characteristics that lead them to enter the field and survive as experts. Scientific researchers, for example, may prefer utilitarian value judgments that can diminish commitment to individual rights. If the average values of the experts differ from the average values of society at large, then the evaluations of the treatment options by the expert group will be systematically biased and deviate from the values that the broader society would use.[16] Thus, not only may individual clinicians and their patients rationally reject treatment protocol recommendations because they reject the values of the protocol writers; the society also may reject the public-policy treatment recommendations of groups of experts if the lay population's values differ from those of the experts.

Some clinicians, clinical researchers, and patients have followed ethicists in concluding that all treatment decisions, including the recommendations in practice guidelines and treatment protocols, necessarily involve value judgments that cannot be derived from the science of medicine. They agree that practice guidelines and treatment protocols necessarily import someone's system of belief and value. Those who accept this conclusion will tolerate clinicians who reject the treatment recommendations of a practice guideline or treatment protocol. If the rejection takes place at the level of the clinician—whose values depart form the values incorporated into the protocol—then the patient is doubly vulnerable. Not only is the patient subject to the personal and professional values of the protocol writers, the patient is also vulnerable to the filtering of the recommendations through the clinician's values. The patient must be informed that treatment recommendations are added by the protocol writers and/or the clinician.

PORT Studies and Other Outcomes Research

Even if clinicians and patients understandably reject recommendations in practice guidelines and treatment protocols because they reject values incorporated into them, many still seem to believe that clinicians and patients ought to accept at least the fact finding in technology assessments. As we have seen, some technology assessments are not so ambitious as to strive to make treatment recommendations, but claim only to report the relevant medical facts. If technology assessment could only report the fact that an intervention has a certain effect, then patients, clinicians, and public-policy makers could impose their externally derived evaluations.

One purported function of some varieties of outcomes research is to provide a consensus of expert medical researchers on the relevant medical facts about a particular medical intervention. This more modest function of technology assessment will admittedly not provide the leverage that some have expected from practice guidelines that provide recommendations. It will not provide any basis for evaluating the facts and, logically, cannot provide any recommendations for treatment interventions. It cannot even supply all the relevant facts; it cannot supply the nonmedical facts necessary in any sound treatment decision. But outcomes research could, according to this more modest view of technology assessment, at least give us a scientifically sound basis for estimating the medical facts.

The original PORT studies focus primarily on outcomes. The announcement of the second round of PORT studies (called PORT-II projects) specifies that the projects will examine the effectiveness or cost-effectiveness for the prevention, diagnosis, treatment, and management of common clinical conditions.[17] They seek to compare two or more distinctly different clinical approaches, asking what the outcomes will be, not necessarily going on to ask which outcomes are worth pursuing. Examples from the first round of PORT studies make clear that fact finding was a major objective. The PORT study on ischemic heart disease, for example, found that the Duke Treadmill Score can identify between one-third and two-thirds of outpatients with chest pain who are at low risk for coronary artery disease (CAD); it found that women are not referred for cardiac catheterization as often as men because of a lower incidence of heart disease rather than because of referral bias against women.[18] Interspersed with these findings are treatment recommendations resembling the practice guidelines already discussed. (One report concluded that the benefits of thrombolytic therapy outweigh the risks of intracranial hemorrhage for most acute myocardial infarction [AMI] patients and that U.S. physicians are unnecessarily reluctant to use thrombolytic therapy.)[19] These surely are value judgments imposed on the data, requiring comparison of the harms of myocardial infarction and stroke to iatrogenic and naturally occurring medical problems. Another PORT study, on prostate cancer, also strays into occasional clinical recommendations, concluding that watchful waiting is a reasonable alternative to invasive treatment for men sixty to seventy-five with localized prostate cancer—a judgment that requires assessment of the psychological anxiety of the wait as well as the alternative costs, something that cannot be gleaned from the scientific study.[20] In the studies' defense, the primary focus was on what most medical scientists would consider to be facts: rates of increase of radical prostatectomy, death rates for alternative treatments for localized prostatectomy, etc.

A major effort at the NIH can be viewed as a variety of outcomes assessment. The series of consensus conferences organized by Office of Medical Applications of Research (OMAR) at the NIH is sometimes presented as striving to develop agreement on the medical facts of certain controversial medical technologies.[21] Consensus conferences differ from AHCPR outcomes research. The former do not conduct their own empirical research on the technologies involved but, rather, assemble a panel of leading experts with relevant technical expertise who present the results of their research. A series of questions is presented to the panel which, after listening to two to three days of testimony from leading researchers, goes into closed session to prepare a consensus on its perception of the relevant facts. In spite of their charge, some consensus panels do not restrict themselves to purely factual matters. Many consensus panels drift or are pressured into clinical and public-policy recommendations.

The series of conferences has covered many major areas of medical technology. Usually the questions put to the panel include a number of important matters that would be perceived by most as questions of fact. The critical-care medicine conference asked, "Is there empirical evidence that intensive care units cause a decrease in patient morbidity and mortality?"[22] The electroconvulsive therapy (ECT) conference asked, "What is the evidence that ECT is effective for patients with specific mental disorders?"[23] The blood cholesterol conference asked, "Will reduction of blood cholesterol levels help prevent coronary heart disease?"[24] But each of the panels is also asked some normative questions that require going far beyond the data: What critical-care intervention should be routinely available? What factors should the physician consider in determining that ECT is appropriate? Under what circumstances should dietary or drug treatment be started to treat blood cholesterol?

Unfortunately, recent developments in the philosophy of science and the philosophy of medicine suggest that even this more modest function for technology assessment may face problems in being value-free. The division of clinical reasoning into major and minor premises relies on what philosophers call the fact/value distinction. Its origins go back at least to David Hume. According to it, facts and values are conceptually distinct, so that it is logically impossible to derive a value from a set of facts. In our case, it is logically impossible to derive the value judgment that a treatment ought to be used from the fact that, if it is used, a certain result is likely to be obtained. The "ought" necessarily comes from a different source than the "is." "Oughts" are imposed on the data from the outside.

But recent thought in the philosophy of science is beginning to question this sharp separation. In particular, it is now widely believed that the doing of science itself necessarily incorporates conceptual and normative judgments that make all scientific propositions dependent on these judgments. Holders of this view claim that all statements that are presented as facts actually would be crafted differently if those articulating the statements had different conceptual and normative commitments.

There was a time when the belief prevailed that science at its best was, at least theoretically, objective and value-free. Observations of facts were the source of knowledge about the external world that provided the foundation for confirming or refuting scientific hypotheses. The work of contemporary philosophers of science, such as Fleck,[25] Kuhn,[26] and Feyerabend,[27] and fellow travelers in the sociology of knowledge, such as Luckmann and Berger[28] and the postmodern critics of Hippocratic medical ethics,[29] hold that theory construction in science and the doing of science are inherently dependent on a system of beliefs and values, a thought collective (Fleck), a paradigm (Kuhn), or a worldview.

The paradigm provides the conceptual system that articulates the metaphysical beliefs about the nature of reality, frames the questions being asked, determines which researchable questions are worth pursuing, provides the criteria for observation, establishes the methods of doing research, selects criteria for end points of research, identifies the way findings are reported, and provides the language by which science is communicated.

Just as the Ptolemaic and Copernican worldviews are incommensurable or the medieval world of faith sees reality differently than the modern world of reason, so the doing of science can be divided into two different enterprises: (1) there are moments of revolutionary science in which one paradigm begins to come apart and is replaced by another, and (2) there are periods of normal science where the basic presuppositions are not questioned and puzzles are solved. When one paradigm replaces another, it is not possible to say that there has been progress, but only that there is a different understanding of the world.

One of the most significant theses of post-Kuhnian philosophy of science is that accounts of the world offered by those in different worlds are incommensurable. Even the same words have different meanings. Recently adjustments have led to a distinction between (1) radical incommensurability and (2) local (or partial) incommensurability. Efforts are also under way to apply the notion of incommensurability to smaller, more local divisions in worldview; so, for example, feminist medical scientists and Orthodox Jewish medical scientists can be said to see the world differently, as do more mainstream secular scientists. They ask different questions, have different criteria for proof, use concepts differently, and select different observations as worth recording and publishing.

These developments have important implications for outcomes research and other work in medical science. According to these theorists, medical scientists will necessarily incorporate their system of beliefs and values into the doing of their scientific research. Any account of reality will be framed by the underlying worldview and value system of the one doing the work. Other scientists with other worldviews would have shaped the problem differently, conducted investigations differently, and ended up with different accounts of the reality they are observing—not necessarily any better or worse accounts, just different. Their accounts will be incommensurable with an account of an apparently similar phenomenon seen from a different paradigm. Anyone doing outcomes research will carry with that research a view of the world that will shape the account. Equally competent scientists with another worldview would have given a different account. Outcomes research will not be able to give a single, definitive description of what the effects of a medical intervention will be.

Imagine a group of medical scientists gathered together in an NIH consensus conference for the purpose of generating a consensus on what the outcome will be of a group of medical interventions. The issue may be the outcome of lumpectomy vs. radical surgery for certain specified breast cancers, whether dental sealants will reduce dental caries in children and by how much, whether nurse-midwife home birth is as safe as in-hospital deliveries under the supervision of an obstetrician. The panel members will not all come up with exactly the same assessments of these apparently factual matters. There will be a distribution of views.

Empirical research supports the claim that scientists with different values will give different accounts of the facts. They will be correlated with the scientist's beliefs and values. These are not to be attributed solely to bias or distortion. They are an inevitable result of the necessary influence of paradigm or worldview on the doing of science. Assuming, for example, that the value distribution of scientists is normally distributed about some mean value perspective, there is no a priori reason to assume that the mean estimate of the facts is the most likely to be correct. Moreover, clinicians and patients will also have a distribution of values, but it may not be around the same mean.

Now the relevant question is what is the correct estimate of the facts for the patient or the lay policy maker to use. Obviously, by definition, these laypeople cannot be expert on the facts. If, however, the experts' estimates of the facts correlate with their value frameworks, the proper estimate of the facts for the layperson might appropriately be the one made by the expert whose values correspond to the layperson's. For their individual health care, it seems reasonable that, assuming all members of the expert group are deemed competent, patients take the estimate of the facts that corresponds with the expert who holds values closest to their own.

For public policy we might be inclined to choose the average view of the experts. But the distribution of the values or worldviews of the experts may not be the same as that of the lay population. Perhaps the correct estimate of the outcomes should be the estimate at the point that corresponds to the average value profile of the lay population.

Conclusions

Effects and benefits must be separated. Benefits are fundamentally not knowable by medical science. Outcomes research cannot tell us what the benefits or harms will be; at best it can tell what the effects are likely to be. Therefore outcomes research cannot tell us how much benefit and harm an intervention is likely to produce or which interventions will produce marginal benefit. Even if we could determine which benefits were marginal, that would not determine which interventions were worth providing. Utility maximizers would opt for maximizing aggregate benefit. Advocates for justice would strive to provide benefits for the worst-off persons even if those benefits were more marginal. Lovers of autonomy would take into account whether the needs of patients were brought about by voluntary lifestyle choices of persons needing medical care.

We might be inclined to revert to a model in which outcomes research will provide "just the facts," but contemporary philosophy of science suggests that this is, in principle, impossible. The system of belief and value of the researcher will inevitably shape the framing of the question, the meaning of the language used, the choice of methods, the identification of observations worth reporting, the statistical end points, and the linguistic structure of the account given. Outcomes research cannot even tell us what the effects of interventions are in a value-free way, let alone what the benefits and harms are.

Thus, there may be reasons why clinicians and patients will resist the recommendations of even the best, most carefully developed practice guidelines and treatment protocols. If those guidelines and protocols necessarily incorporate values that may not be those of the clinician or patient, one option could be for the user of the guideline to discount them and adjust them for a preferred value framework. To reach this goal, guideline users would have to distill the factual claims about what the outcomes of the interventions will be; for example, they might more directly turn to outcomes research. But if they do, even here the facts claims will have to be seen as reflecting conceptual and normative commitments that they may not share. Rational consumers of technology assessments, both practice guidelines and outcomes research, will have to take into account that technology assessment necessarily incorporates value judgments and that if the developers of these assessments had different systems of belief and value, they would have articulated their guidelines and outcomes reports differently. Technology assessment is necessarily a value-laden enterprise.

NOTES

1. The very term "manage" is controversial. It is used repeatedly in technology assessment, particularly the AHCPR *Clinical Practice Guidelines*, which use the term in many of their titles. See such titles as *Management of Cataract in Adults* and *Diagnosing and Managing Unstable Angina*. The imagery of managing a human being is considered offensive by some critics of contemporary health care who believe it implies a paternalism, a lack of respect for patient autonomy, yet the writers of these guidelines appear not to grasp this controversy. It is pejorative in the same way that "girl" is when used to refer to adult females, or "boy" to refer to African-American adult males. To these critics management is something one does to a commodities portfolio or a group of subordinate employees.

2. Robert M. Veatch, "Values in Routine Medical Decisions," and "The Concept of 'Medical Indications,'" in *The Patient-Physician Relation: The Patient as Partner, Part 2* (Bloomington: Indiana University Press, 1991), pp. 47–62.

3. "PORT Researchers Discuss Treatment Options and Use of Serum PSA Screening to Detect Prostate Cancer," *Research Activities,* no. 181 (January 1995): 5.

4. Office for Medical Applications of Research, *Participants' Guide to Consensus Development Conferences* (Bethesda: U.S. Department of Health, Education, and Welfare, [n.d.]), p. 1.

5. NIH Consensus Development Panel on Gallstones and Laparoscopic Cholecystectomy, "Gallstones and Laparoscopic Cholecystectomy," *JAMA* 269, no. 8 (1993): 1018–24 at 1021.

6. NIH Consensus Development Panel on Gallstones, "Gallstones," p. 1019.

7. National Institutes of Health, "Consensus Development Conference Statement: Dental Sealants in the Prevention of Tooth Decay," *Journal of Dental Education* 48, Supplement (February 1984): 126–31.

8. Robert F. Nease et al., "Variation in Patient Utilities for Outcomes of the Management of Chronic Stable Angina: Implications for Clinical Practice Guidelines," *JAMA* 273, no. 15 (1995): 1185–90.

9. AHCPR, *Management of Cataract in Adults,* Number 4 (Washington, D.C.: U.S. Government Printing Office, 1994).

10. AHCPR, *Management of Cancer Pain: Adults,* Number 9 (Washington, D.C.: U.S. Government Printing Office, 1994), pp. 8–9.

11. AHCPR, *Depression in Primary Care; Detection, Diagnosis, and Treatment*, Number 5 (Washington, D.C.: U.S. Government Printing Office, 1993), p. 6.

12. AHCPR, *Managing Otitis Media with Effusion in Young Children*, Number 12 (Washington, D.C.: U.S. Government Printing Office, 1994), p. 6.

13. AHCPR, *Managing Otitis Media,* p. 5.

14. Robert M. Veatch, "Abandoning Informed Consent," *Hastings Center Report* 25, no. 2 (1995): 5–12.

15. Judith Areen, "The Legal Status of Consent Obtained from Families of Adult Patients to Withhold or Withdraw Treatment," *Journal of the American Medical Association* 258, no. 2 (1987): 229–35; Robert M. Veatch, "Limits of Guardian Treatment Refusal: A Reasonableness Standard," *American Journal of Law and Medicine* 9, no. 4 (1984): 427–68.

16. For a more complete discussion of the problem of mismatch between the consensus values of the lay and expert groups see Robert M. Veatch, "Consensus of Expertise: The Role of Consensus of Experts in Formulating Public Policy and Estimating Facts," *Journal of Medicine and Philosophy* 16 (1991): 427–45.

17. "AHCPR Invites Proposals for PORT-II Projects," *Research Activities,* no. 167 (August 1993): 15.

18. "Ischemic Heart Disease PORT Publishes Latest Findings," *Research Activities,* no. 176 (July 1994): 6–7.

19. "Ischemic Heart Disease PORT," p. 6.

20. C. Fleming et al., "A Decision Analysis of Alternative Treatment Strategies for Clinically Localized Prostate Cancer," *JAMA,* 269, no. 20 (1993): 2650–8.

21. See NIH, Office for Medical Applications of Research, *Participants' Guide to Consensus Development Conferences* (Bethesda: U.S. Department of Health, Education, and Welfare, [n.d.]), where one of the stated criteria for the conferences is that "the topic should be resolvable on technical grounds and the outcome should not depend mainly on value judgments of panelists."

22. NIH Consensus Development Panel, "Critical Care Medicine," *JAMA* 250, no. 6 (1983): 798–804.

23. Office for Medical Applications of Research, "Electroconvulsive Therapy," *JAMA* 254, no. 15 (1985): 2103–8.

24. Office for Medical Applications of Research, "Lowering Blood Cholesterol to Prevent Heart Disease," *JAMA* 253, no. 14 (1985): 2080–6.

25. Ludwig Fleck, *Genesis and Development of a Scientific Fact,* ed. Thaddeus J. Trenn and Robert K. Merton, transl. Fred Bradley and Thaddeus J. Trenn (Chicago: University of Chicago Press, 1979).

26. Thomas S. Kuhn, *The Structure of Scientific Revolutions* (Chicago: University of Chicago Press, 1962).

27. P. K. Feyerabend, *Realism, Rationalism, and Scientific Method: Philosophical Papers, Volume 1* (Cambridge: Cambridge University Press, 1981).

28. Peter L. Berger and Thomas Luckmann, *The Social Construction of Reality* (New York: Doubleday, 1967).

29. Robert M. Veatch, *Value-Freedom in Science and Technology* (Missoula, Mont.: Scholars Press, 1976).

JAMES LINDEMANN NELSON

Clinical Judgment versus Outcomes Research?

A Tale of Two Health Care Centers

At a major integrated health care system in the eastern Midwest, many practitioners don't use tissue plasminogen activator (t-PA) despite the evidence of superior outcomes as attested to by the GUSTO II trials. In part this is due to logistics—many heart patients present at satellite clinics not equipped to use this clot buster. Yet most other practitioners in the system, not so restricted, also favor streptokinase. When pressed as to the reasons for their decision, they often say that the GUSTO data are not "clinically meaningful," at least for their populations.[1]

At a distinguished community hospital in New York State, the practice pattern is different. There t-PA is used virtually all the time. But the hospital's cardiologists say that they regard streptokinase as a perfectly legitimate therapeutic option. Despite the evidence derived from outcomes research, they were unanimous in saying that they would resist any attempts to influence a physician to use t-PA against his or her better judgment.[2]

The moral I want to abstract from these stories is that at least some clinicians regard thoughtful decisions made by working physicians—what I will henceforth call "clinical judgment"—as an appropriate counterweight to the apparent direction of outcomes research. In the first case, this may not seem surprising: the physicians in question do not use t-PA, and hence they are under considerable pressure to argue that electing other anticoagulants is perfectly reasonable. But the second case is perhaps more striking. These physicians all defended using other anticoagulants counterfactually, so to speak, and this despite the fact that the community standard of practice runs smack in the face of using anything other than t-PA. Furthermore, the cardiologists all regarded the research standards involved in the GUSTO II studies to be impeccable and definitive; given the scope and outcome of that trial, the cardiologists thought it extremely unlikely that any further, more authoritative work would be done on the question, and hence GUSTO II is the absolute last word on the subject.

Why Judgment Matters

What is it about physician judgment that makes experienced and well-placed clinicians defer to it—at least in principle—even in the face of widespread community practice to the contrary and countervailing outcomes research of the highest quality? One possible explanation is psychological or sociological in orientation: roughly put, that the exercise of sophisticated judgment is one of the sources of the special authority of physicians in the eyes of their patients, as well as a source of the special satisfaction of medical practice. In other words, when Hippocrates tells us that "life is short and the art long, the occasion fleeting, experiment perilous, judgment difficult," he's not wringing his hands. Rather, he's sketching a place distinctly inviting to those inclined to strive to do something that is both very significant and very difficult and that, deservedly, should command the respect of the laity. The difficulty with outcomes research–based practice guidelines that have any bite to them, then, at least in this view, is that they undermine the exercise of clinical judgment as a source of physician authority and satisfaction.

But even if there is anything to this hypothesis, it constitutes, as it stands, only an explanation, not a justification, of physician reluctance to allow outcomes research pride of place over clinical judgment. It might be more satisfying for doctors to be the purveyors of an arcane expertise of their own rather than the servants of expert systems, votaries in the temple of outcomes research, but if practice guidelines based on such research get us more health for less money, then they are going to have to lump it.

Furthermore, even in a kind of medical practice that paid more thorough and systematic attention to outcomes research–based evidence, there would still be plenty of scope for the exercise of physicianly skill. There is a sense of "judgment" in which its exercise is ineliminable as a matter of logic; as Kant and Wittgenstein have shown, the application of general rules to specific cases will always involve an ability that is not itself rule-governed, on pain of infinite regress. (If every application of a rule to a concrete situation involved the invocation of another rule, then a third rule would be required to apply the second, a fourth for the guidance of the third, and so on.)[3] But as this result holds so generally—not only for making tough medical calls, but, for example, for being able to apply the concept "chair" to those objects in the world that fall into its extension—it might not seem very exciting. What will always be needed is not simply judgment but expert judgment, complex judgment, satisfying judgment, "judgment difficult." Guidelines based on outcomes research will have to be adjusted to particular cases, clinicians will have to be canny about when to appeal the verdicts of economically enforced guidelines and when not to, and they may even be able to use the guidelines to reinforce their own particular perception of what is significant about cases. If guidelines offer a well-grounded view about what is standard, then against this backdrop interesting variations may stand out more clearly and hence be more often perceived, and beneficially affect both therapy and future research.

But there is a more interesting, more direct assault on outcomes research than that reliance on its results might make being a physician less interesting and less authoritative. It is more directly epistemic, where the underlying theme is not that clinical judgment is more fun to do than is applying algorithms but that clinical judgment responds to sources of knowledge that outcomes research misses. In other words, outcomes research makes a claim to a kind of epistemic hegemony that it can't support in its own terms: practice guided primarily by outcomes data is not necessarily going to be practice that more efficiently achieves good outcomes.

This thesis—or one very much like it—has already been defended very ably by Sandra Tanenbaum.[4] She has argued that outcomes research is all very well in its place but that its place is determined by such matters as concerns about the projectibility of the clinically relevant traits of the patients used in its studies, by the taint left by investigator bias and the self-interest of funders. More interestingly still, she has pointed out that the traditional forms of epistemic warrant for what doctors believe and do come from a philosophy of medicine distinct from that of outcomes researchers.

Doctors, as Tanenbaum sees it, typically are realists and determinists: that is, they think that patient symptoms are typically caused by some real set of properties within bodies and that we can come to understand those properties and how and why they are dysfunctional. On the basis of the model of what's wrong that undergirds the story the physician tells to make sense to herself and her patient of what's going on, reasonable responses can be crafted. Outcomes researchers, on the other hand, assume a different epistemic stance. They are probabilists and empiricists. In her portrayal, they don't really care why things happen as they happen, and they don't build models. What they are good at is locating correlations. They know, for example, what the percentages are that unopposed estrogen treatment will reduce chances of congestive heart disease in postmenopausal women without uteruses and without family history of breast cancer, and what that is likely to mean to women—at least to women similar in all relevant respects to their study population—in terms of their longevity. Qua outcomes researchers, anyway, they don't know why it works the way it does, and they don't want to know.

Tanenbaum points out that this sort of thing is problematic for patients for whom things don't work out as the study predicts or who fall outside the parameters of the study population. Suppose, for example, that a woman who doesn't have a uterus but does have a family history of breast cancer comes to a physician. Is unopposed ERT a good bet for her? Outcomes studies don't speak to this issue directly. On the other hand, realist models of pathophysiology, generated by bench science and informed by practitioner experience, do provide the doctor with grounds for saying useful things in such occasions.

How is Tanenbaum's challenge to be assessed? The epistemic infelicities of outcomes research—its generalization, its failure to suggest models to support inferences when doctors run into statistical outliers—are real and worrisome. But they can probably be met roughly point for point if we turn critical eyes on the realist-determinist model. There are certainly lacunae, lapses, and limits to outcomes research. But bench science has its own limitation and its own outliers. The Wennburg small-area practice variation studies suggest that, in use, either realist-determinist doctors draw different inferences from the same kinds of interaction of data and model or there are confounding influences on diagnosis and choice of therapy.

There is, no doubt, a long story to be told here, and one potentially of great interest. But for now, I am going to assume that, strictly on a priori grounds, one might as well say that this dispute looks something like a wash— there are limitations to both ways of forming medical decisions. This in itself is a significant result that ought to have some ability to temper any single-minded zealotry about outcomes research. But the deeper moral many might draw is that we ought to just get even more a posteriori and systematic about the issue. That is, let's see if various kinds of reliance on outcomes measures make a difference and, insofar as they do, make adjustments in practice accordingly.

Taking Judgment Seriously

Is there reason to shy away from even this measured conclusion? Possibly. Clinician judgment is not distinguished from outcomes research and practice guidelines simply in terms of the realist/empiricist split, at least as it is understood in the ontological sense that Tanenbaum stresses. Doctors also are *epistemological* realists, antiskeptics—that is, they see the real world as one for which human modes of thought are well suited. It isn't just that the truth is there. It's that human beings are tolerably good at figuring it out, and in a lot of different ways. Some such epistemological view seems required to make sense of the fact that doctors are inclined to rely a great deal on the notion of a kind of judgment that doesn't seem strictly rule-governed or rule-guided, no matter whether those rules are generated from outcomes research or basic science, but that yet somehow manage to intuit the truth.

So there is a source of clinical authority relied upon by physicians that would resist the hegemony of the statistical, even if some form of it were found to outperform realist models. This sort of thing is often talked of in terms of sensitivity to irreducible particulars or to intuitions. But neither of these ideas is going to cut much ice with people who are devotees of outcomes research *über alles*. Something has to be done to cash out the epistemic bona fides of such appeals.

There is reason to believe that expert judgment in many domains is not reducible to explicit rules and rule following. There are vivid examples of this in chess. In chess, there are rules for moving pieces, of course, and even rules, or counsels of strategy, that orient you to where you should be moving them, plus a lot of necessary memorization of standard openings, replies, and end games. The novice learns these rules—for example, learns to be wary of weakening her pawn structure—and the more advanced, more truly competent player knows them better and more of them. But the true expert—the master-level chess player—isn't just an even more competent player, knowing even more rules even better. There seems to be something entirely different going on in the master's head. This is illustrated by the fact that masters can play extremely fast without significantly lowering the quality of their play. In a rather vivid little experiment reported by Hubert Dreyfus,[5] a chess master played speed chess against a fellow master while continually solving addition problems, a new one presented every few seconds. According to Dreyfus, the master produced unbroken streams of fluent and strategically deep chess. It seems that something other than deliberation according to rules was going on.

It would be nice to know what that something was, of course. It isn't exactly a nouveau phenomenon: Aristotle seemed to have something similar in mind in the *Nichomachean Ethics* when discussing the activity of experts in the domain of ethical judgment. In that sphere, judgment, he thought, is not an activity governed by general rules but, rather, one that is sensitive to the special features of a particular situation. It can be learned, not in any rote fashion but rather by imitation of those who already possess it. What it is that is learned in this fashion, however, is not described.[6]

But even if we admit that there is something to the judgment of experts that is not altogether captured by rules, unless we can get clearer about what that something is, then we won't be able to assess what's going on in expert judgment now vis-à-vis what it could be like if it were more circumscribed or more thoroughly informed by rules. After all, while it may be clear that the expertise of the chess master is not modeled in any realistic sense by chess-playing computers, it is noteworthy that computers can now give even the highest-rated masters a very tough game. So even if there is an epistemically respectable source of expert judgment possessed by (some? most?) clinicians, it behooves us to get clearer about what it might be, because it is still very reasonable to try to understand its limits as well.

The chess analog should not, of course, be pressed too hard, but exploration of this kind tends to be driven by analogs, for better or worse. In an interesting paper by Marx Wartofsky,[7] clinical judgment—he's concentrating particularly on diagnostic skill—is likened to the complex cognitive-affective procedures involved in getting the point of a joke. For example, you may have heard that Bill Clinton went fishing with the pope the other day, and the pope's miter was blown off his head and into the water. "Not to worry, Your Holiness," said Bill, and he hopped out of the boat, strolled across the water, retrieved the symbol of the pope's office, and jogged back to the boat. On-shore press captured this event on film, and the headline in the next morning's *Times* read, "CLINTON CAN'T SWIM."

Wartofsky's point seems to be that to get a joke, one has to be able to draw upon a vast reserve of knowledge. Human beings are able to appreciate relationships among sets of data, and that appreciation draws on a rich cultural backdrop. One needs to know a lot about contemporary American culture to get the point of this joke, to appreciate the connections that give it its humor. Analogously, you need to know a lot to be a good diagnostician, and not just a lot about medicine, or so I take Wartofsky to be saying—you just need to know a lot. A diagnostician, for example, has at her beck and call, in some not fully conscious way, what she has imbibed from a lifetime's immersion in an entire culture. This becomes a rich source of metaphor, analogy, comparison, and patterns that may somehow give rise to an insight that relates medical variables in rich and significant new ways.

Other people who have written about the way in which expert judgment is qualitatively different from merely competent decision making also stress an element in Wartofsky's account that might be called "pattern recognition"; Tanenbaum, for instance, speaks of the clinician's "grasp of a meaningful medical whole."[8] When you take smart and highly enculturated people and give them a large amount of experience in a particular domain—particularly experience that is highly emotionally loaded—they develop facility at recognizing salient patterns.

Now suppose, at least for sake of argument, we accept that there are forms of expert judgment that can't be modeled by algorithms or rules or guidelines of other sorts, and suppose we even accept that clinical judgment may be included among them. As the example of chess computers outplaying people who have this kind of expert judgment indicates, it does not follow that clinical judgment driven in such ways is superior to good outcomes research. It does not, for example, follow that anyone who resists the GUSTO study and uses streptokinase is to be supported. At least if we abstract from cost-benefit concerns, it may well be the case that such a policy is poor medicine, below what should be regarded as a standard of care.

Proponents of clinical judgment have been embarrassed by studies that have indicated that, in those cases where a formula has been developed that relates symptoms to disease, the formula outperforms the diagnostic accuracy of experienced clinicians by significant margins.[9] This has indicated to some observers that, while clinical judgment is not exactly bogus, neither is it always, or even all that often, reliable. They conclude that what we need are more of those powerful diagnostic formulae, as well as their therapeutic analogs, and outcomes research would seem to be a good way of developing them. But this is too quick an inference. Even if formulae outperform experienced clinicians in the aggregate, it does not outperform all clinicians: some are especially good at diagnosis and do better than the formulae.

What this suggests is that a program of research that was anxious to find out what works and what doesn't ought to look not only at statistical research but at ethnology, so to speak, as well. What is it that makes the superior clinician a superior clinician? Can her patterns of perception, judgment, and action be better understood and generalized to others?

Designing Guidelines as if Judgment Mattered

All this suggests two recommendations, one concerning the use of practice guidelines, the second, directions for further investigation. First, practice guidelines coming out of outcomes research should be couched in ways that recognize that clinical judgment is an indispensable part of the practice of medicine. They should acknowledge that clinical judgment has a claim to respect, which practice variations can't altogether undermine. Clinical judgment is—or, at least, may be in favored instances—founded in a ubiquitous, if somewhat mysterious, kind of reliable epistemic capacity. Further, doctors are, with some justification, proud of their abilities in this regard and are unlikely to cotton up willingly to approaches that seem too foreign and too disrespectful of existing patterns.

Second, inquiry should be conducted directly into the phenomenon of expert judgment. This is an inquiry that should have a conceptual dimension, a cognitive-psychology and cognitive-science dimension, and an ethnographic dimension. There is a richer story to be told about "judgment difficult" than has yet been told. Aristotle, Kant, and Wittgenstein have traced out some of its contours, but the whole area is really too important not to keep thinking hard about.[10]

NOTES

1. Data drawn from interviews conducted by staff of The Hastings Center's project "Technology Assessment: Uses, Context, and Interpretation," fall 1994.

2. Based on interviews conducted by staff of The Hastings Center's project "Technology Assessment: Uses, Context, and Interpretation," summer 1994.

3. For Kant's views, see the *Critique of Pure Reason*, 1781 edition, 134. For Wittgenstein, the *Philosophical Investigations*, part II, section xi.

4. Sandra Tanenbaum, "Outcomes Research in Medical Practice: Signposts and Speedbumps in the Moral Terrain," presented at The Hastings Center, Technology Assessment Meeting, December 13–14, 1993.

5. Hubert Dreyfus and Stuart Dreyfus, "What Is Morality? A Phenomenological Account of the Development of Ethical Expertise," in *Universalism vs. Communitarianism*, David Rasmussen, ed. (Cambridge: MIT Press, 1990).

6. Aristotle, *Nichomachean Ethics*, 1104a9; I am indebted to Charles Larmore's discussion in *Patterns of Moral Complexity* (Cambridge: Cambridge University Press, 1987), chapter 1.

7. Marx Wartofsky, "Clinical Judgment, Expert Programs, and Cognitive Style: A Counter-Essay in the Logic of Diagnosis," *Journal of Medicine and Philosophy* 11 (1986): 81–92.

8. Tanenbaum, "Outcomes Research," p. 5.

9. Michael Scriven, "Clinical Judgment," in *Clinical Judgment: A Critical Appraisal*, H. Tristram Engelhardt et al., eds. (Dordrecht, Netherlands: Reidel, 1979), pp. 3–16.

10. I much appreciate the reaction of many of the participants in The Hastings Center project "Technology Assessment: Uses, Context, and Interpretation" to this work. It is also a pleasure to acknowledge the support of the AHCPR.

Sandra J. Tanenbaum

Say the Right Thing: Communication and Physician Accountability in the Era of Medical Outcomes

Introduction

Although health care reform remains unconsummated, there exists broad consensus—among congressional allies and enemies, interest groups of every stripe, and otherwise nonaligned members of the public—that the U.S. health care system is a wasteful one. Its substantial expenditures are patently misguided, yet it is unaccountable to payers and patients for how much is spent and on what.[1] In fact, a far-flung movement for "assessment and accountability" on the part of providers (and especially physicians, on whom this paper is focused) has been designated the "third revolution in medical care."[2] Virtually every recent proposal for reform posits informed consumers, choosing among competing providers, who in turn offer assessment of, and accountability for, the cost and quality of health services.

Oddly enough, the definition of "accountability" in this health care context is mostly unspecified. To be sure, the term always implies answering for—that is, bearing the consequences of—one's actions. In our market-based health care system, this usually means bearing the economic consequences of consumer dissatisfaction, and because health care is not an ordinary consumer good, "consumer" dissatisfaction may affect the patient himself, his payer, or the responsible regulatory agent. In any case, accountability for health care typically means the measurement of some aspect of care against a preconceived standard. Promotion of appropriate standards comprising medical outcomes has recently been most influential. It is sometimes referred to as the "outcomes movement."[3]

Here I offer a critique of the outcomes movement and of the applied-science model of medical practice on which it rests. More to the point, however, this paper argues that the dominant definition of "accountability" is needlessly limited and even counterproductive. The "accountability" of recent health policy developments is not the "obligation to make an accounting" but something more like an "obligation to endure second- or third-party sanction for violation of that party's standard." The accountable provider does not engage in the process of communicating her account; rather, an overt behavior—hers or her patient's—is measured and judged against some fixed and often statistical criterion.[4] The losses from adopting this latter definition are not trivial: they include, as will be elaborated, a false certainty about partial knowledge and the incapacity to integrate plural knowledge and values into a meaningful whole, especially at the level of the individual patient but also for the policy-making process.

In this paper, I propose an alternative conception of accountability in health care, one more closely modeled on the original meaning of the word. "Communicative accountability," as I refer to it, derives from a humanist view of medical practice, from my earlier work on the outcomes movement, and from Jürgen Habermas's treatment of communicative action.[5] In defining "communicative accountability," I follow roughly Habermas's three-part delineation of communicative action (although I regard his work as a resource for, and not a defense of, my own) and, at each juncture, transpose an element of Habermas's schema to describe the special case of physician accountability to patients. This creates a clear contrast to the more common conception of accountability, which I will call "standard accountability," and one that is ultimately no more impractical for its philosophical roots.

Part One: The Logic of Communicative Accountability

At its simplest, communicative accountability in health care emphasizes the making of an account, that is, the communicated accounting for medical care (including its outcomes). In contrast, the dominant conception dispenses with the accounting process, apparently confounding a behavioral standard met with an actual accounting made. This seems to be the case whether the standard is the patient's, physician's, or someone else's and whether the evidence of its having been met is case-specific or in the aggregate. Whereas communicative accountability requires physicians to review, explain, and justify individual acts in context, standard accountability emphasizes the correspondence of physician behavior, often in the quantitative abstract, to some predetermined criterion.

Communicative accountability assumes that clinical medicine is essentially a relationship between a single patient and a physician. This is not to deny the contribution of public health to average lifespan, nor to overlook the role of nurses and technicians in hospital care, nor to minimize the health maintenance potential of a supportive household, nor even to privilege medical entitlements over housing and environmental programs. Neither is it to ignore the many nonclinical influences on physicians' and patients' behavior in the clinic. It is only to maintain that medical practice per se is a relationship between two complex human beings and that the logic of physician accountability (and, by extension, the accountability of clinicians generally) should be modeled on what we know of that relationship.

This model also builds on the philosophical treatment of human communication generally and specifically on Habermas's description of a three-part communicative act. Habermas's schema both characterizes existing physician-patient relationships[6] and suggests a realistic framework for enhancing accountability in health care. For if accountability is the obligation to make an accounting—rather than the sanctionability of not exhibiting, or eliciting, behavior that conforms to some standard—then it refers, primarily, to a communicative act. It follows that greater accountability can only issue from better communication, not the more efficient exchange of more effective information but human communication in all its aspects.

Habermas has identified three functions, usually present in the same utterance, that distinguish human communication: "to represent something in the world, to express the speaker's intentions, and to establish legitimate interpersonal relations."[7] The speaker, correspondingly, makes three claims as to the validity of his utterance, to "truth, truthfulness, and rightness" respectively.[8] Following Habermas, I propose to schematize the physician's account—as a species of physician-patient communication—as follows: it comprises the physician's representation of the medical problem and preferred solutions, including relevant medical history and history of the doctor-patient relationship; the physician's statement of the limits of that representation, including disputed science, personal uncertainties, and past mistakes; and the physician's participation, with the patient, in a relationship where disclosure, challenge, and rerepresentation are valued. The accountability criteria may similarly be compared to Habermas's validity claims: a physician is more accountable, that is, he makes a more valid accounting, to the extent that his representation of the case is knowledgeable—that is, medically correct and current as well as cognizant of important particularities to this patient; that it includes a frank assessment of what is known in relation to what is unknown and that this assessment includes the physician's self-representation as imperfect knower; and that it issues from and creates a patient-physician relationship with the time, mutual respect, and collaborative repertoire for negotiating, and acting on, the meanings of illness and care.

There are two basic justifications for communicative accountability in medical care. The second—that communicative accountability avoids many of the specific weaknesses of standard accountability—will be elaborated in the next section. The first, however, is that as in the act of "accounting," clinical medicine is primarily communicative. In spite of the technological intensity of contemporary health care, the basic unit of medical practice is still one physician and one patient talking to one another. Even scholars working in divergent intellectual traditions repeatedly observe the significance of communication to medical practice.

A recent review of what might be called positivist social-psychological literature notes that physician-patient communication is increasingly the subject of scholarly investigation, perhaps because communication "can be seen as the main ingredient in medical care."[9] Among the specific findings cited in the review (of 112 entries published since 1979) were that physician information giving and lengthier physician-patient interviews were positively related to patient satisfaction. In one study, patient compliance with treatment regimens was positively associated with "sharing opinions" with the physician and "patient knowledge about illness"; in another, the length of time physicians spend relating medical information and opinions was found to predict patients' levels of understanding of what they were told.

From a very different perspective—that of qualitative social science and literary studies—physician-patient communication is construed in part as the telling of stories.[10] Mary-Jo Delvecchio Good identifies "clinical narratives" as a specific area of physician competence and the means by which "treatment decisions and the experience of disease may be placed within the overall life course of patients."[11] These narratives are essential to patient evaluation and require the communicative skills of a reader or writer of stories: "To respect language, to adopt alien points of view, to integrate isolated phenomena (be they physical findings or metaphors) so that they suggest meaning, to organize events into a narrative that leads toward their conclusion, and to understand one story in the context of other stories by the same teller."[12]

Whatever the outcome, the experience of illness is meaningful for both patient and physician. At the very least, diagnosis and treatment require the latter to make sense of a patient's signs and symptoms. Moreover, because the patient too interprets this illness, the physician ideally augments a professional interpretation with the patient's and so comes to understand the illness from within the patient's own system of meaning.[13] Physician and patient may be said to negotiate diagnosis and treatment, telling and retelling the illness story until there is a version both can abide.[14] Narrative collaboration should not be confused with the strategic negotiations of a consumerist model. The point is not to satisfy preexisting preferences but to participate in the determination—and realization—of what is wrong and how to set it right.

Bioethicists also point up the singular importance of physician-patient communication. For example, clinical narrative is considered desirable in part because it allows the physician, who will manage eventual ethical quandaries, "to surmise the texture of a patient's life in all its moral complexity."[15] Morreim argues the point more emphatically in her consideration of medical ethics under the new medical economics: "Probably more than anything else, the revised ethic of medicine must emphasize communication"[16] so that physicians may share with their patients the new complexity of the medical encounter and patients in turn may be more responsible for their own care. What is required, according to Morreim, is "careful conversation,"[17] and I would offer her accountability criteria as a working definition for the physician's careful account.

Part Two: Contrasting Standard and Communicative Accountabilities

Communicative accountability is clearly rendered by contrasting it to standard accountability, which, as previously noted, emphasizes sanctionable behavior measured against some criterion. Medical outcomes, such as mortality and functionality, are often the preferred standard, and there exists a veritable "outcomes movement," whose purpose is to create accountable health care by determining what works in medicine and holding providers to that standard.[18] The outcomes movement responds primarily to research findings of large, and "unexplained," variation in rates of health services utilization across ostensibly similar geographic regions. Researchers argue that physician uncertainty accounts for these disparities and that outcome studies—statistical analyses of large health care databases—will achieve the requisite clinical certainty.[19] Congress, among others, has found the logic of the movement persuasive. In 1989 the Agency for Health Care Policy and Research (AHCPR) was legislated into existence to conduct outcomes research specifically and to implement research findings through the issuance of practice guidelines. Before newly powerful Congressional budget cutters set their sights on the agency in the spring of 1995, AHCPR's budget had grown from an original $97 million to $173 million in FY 1995.[20] During the health care reform debate of 1993–1994, every major legislative proposal would have provided for expanded outcomes research.[21]

Although outcomes research need not generate practice guidelines nor other standards and although standards may derive from consensus rather than research, AHCPR's coupling of outcomes research and practice guidelines was not incidental. Rather, both outcomes research and practice guidelines conceive medicine as applied science and therefore the best medicine as the closest alignment of physician behavior with scientific fact. Outcomes research seeks to provide physicians with new and powerful facts, and whereas practice guidelines are but a single means of dissemination, they are arguably the most effective one. By expressing research findings as rules of conduct—as a set of standardized behaviors—guidelines prevent slippage between what researchers know and what practitioners do.

Outcomes measurement is a fairly recent variation on standard accountability. Utilization reviewers, in contrast, have for many years enforced physicians' standard accountability to health care payers and managers. Tallying resources utilized against care delivered at a moment in time and shaping physician behavior toward some ideal, by sanctioning deviation from length-of-stay standards or average rates of referral to specialists, for example, utilization review is a clear-cut exercise in standard accountability and, as such, is logically compatible with more erudite outcomes research–based practice guidelines. In both cases, physicians are deemed to be practicing accountable medicine when behavior is measured against, and shaped to, quantifiable criteria. Although standard accountability presents both practical and conceptual difficulties (some of which will be discussed here), most analysts who grant these shortcomings insist that the only alternative is rampant ignorance, limitless health care spending, and patient exploitation. Few alternative accountability models have been set forth.

To distinguish the workings of standard accountability from those of the communicative alternative, I offer the following simplified example of an elderly woman, with back and leg pain resulting from spinal stenosis, who visits her primary care physician for pain relief and potential treatment. Of what does this physician's accountability consist? Under the dictates of standard accountability, the physician will avail himself of the outcomes literature on this condition, consult existing guidelines for its management, and/or simply defer to the practice policies established in his practice setting or by the patient's insurer. If the physician discovers that there is no compelling reason to take one course over another, he will offer the patient a choice among the several options, providing, in conversation or in writing, summary statistical evidence of the effectiveness, and hopefully the side effects, of each. Because one of the options is likely to be surgery, the primary care physician will refer the patient to one or two neurosurgeons, with whom she may schedule consultative visits. Ideally, the primary care physician will be able to pass along evaluative data on each of the surgeons—procedure-specific mortality and complication rates and perhaps patient satisfaction data, at least at the procedure or hospital level. If not, the patient will be urged to secure these data at the consultative visit. The interpersonal relationship between the primary care physician and the patient will, with any luck, be commodious for both. Its purpose, however, is to achieve medical effectiveness and so to exchange the information on which that effectiveness depends. The physician's account is a precis of the relevant data, his justificatory framework the "best" science, under which all physician-patient relationships are subsumed.

The communicative version of physician accountability has many of the same elements but positions—and values—them differently. The primary accountability of the primary care physician is to the patient, and it is the three-part accountability of communicative action. First, the physician assembles his knowledge of spinal stenosis, which knowledge comprises varieties of medical science and lore, professional expertise and experience, and thus includes but is not reducible to outcomes research and practice guidelines. He probably organizes the outcomes material around his mechanistic understanding of spinal disorders and their amelioration; he is likely to have to reconcile conflicting guidelines and compensate for incomplete information with reference not only to anatomy and physiology but to his own past experiences with spinal stenosis patients. The accountable physician then particularizes his understanding of the illness with his knowledge of the patient. Especially if he has been her primary care physician for some time, her stenosis presents itself in a context thick with medical and personal history (of heart disease and widowhood, for example; her particular preferences for mobility, comfort, predictability; a high tolerance for pain but not for immobility; a general willingness to take a risk) and a set of current and future circumstances (the necessity of exercise for her cardiac care, her son's insistence that she find supported housing as she becomes romantically involved with the widower next door) in which the patient is likely to experience her illness.

As regards the second and third elements of communicative accountability, the physician communicates his multifaceted preliminary account to his patient with careful attention to how good an account he thinks it is and why. He recognizes the weaknesses of the relevant science (the studies do not support a clear conclusion, for example), his biases (against invasive procedures in the elderly perhaps), uncertainties (about her borderline or contradictory test results), and intuitions (about her as a surgical patient); he apprises the patient of how someone else (a surgeon, say) might portray her situation differently. As above, the physician provides information and invites the patient to determine her course, but uncertainty is readily admitted to and the very terms of evaluation are culled from the patient's own discussion of her illness, life, and values. When has she previously faced a decision of this kind? What did she decide, and how did it work out? How does she imagine dealing with her back problems in the future? Finally, the physician-patient relationship accommodates and is a function of this communication. It features sufficiently long and frequent visits or telephone calls, it cultivates mutual respect, and it develops a collaborative routine that surpasses, say, a decision tree for choosing and abiding a course of stenosis treatment.

Physician-patient collaboration in the current health care environment must also include the physician's disclosure of institutional influences on his practice. The elderly stenosis patient is likely a Medicare beneficiary, so the physician will bring to their collaborative accounting the effect of Medicare reimbursement policy on her choice of surgery over physical therapy, for example. If in some other case the physician serves a capitated plan, collaboration requires that he disclose the incentives to keep a patient's surgical referrals to a minimum. Ultimately, the physician may or may not recommend a surgical consultation, the elderly woman may or may not decide to undergo surgery, and either or both of them may later believe that the wrong decision was made. The accountability of the physician is not thereby compromised, however; being accountable is not the same as making the decision one would make in retrospect. Communicative accountability indeed emphasizes a capacity for self-correction, because in the daily practice of clinical medicine, almost everyone learns from experience.

Evidence, Fact, and Truth

As we turn specifically to the three functions of a physician's account, it should be noted that one of the strongest arguments for standard accountability is that it subjects physician behavior to the discipline of facts or "evidence." By "facts" is usually meant the findings of probabilistic research studies; indeed these studies are widely considered the foundation of a new, more scientific medicine. In a statement characteristic of this perspective, Davidoff et al. hold that "increasing realization of the power of probabilistic reasoning has now shifted us from an older anecdotal to a new epidemiologic standard . . . , thus 'raising the bar' for the acceptable level of etiologic and diagnostic evidence."[22] In other words, new methods have brought us new knowledge— better knowledge—and the best medicine will adhere as closely as possible to it. Claims for this knowledge are substantial. Although a single study may "provide the truth," the "whole truth may require a synthesis of the evidence from all the best studies."[23]

The nature of medical truth is not, however, and has never been, something about which all medical thinkers agree. Philosophers and historians of medicine identify[24] and physicians themselves attest to[25] two major and sometimes antagonistic schools of medical thought. The medical realist, on the one hand, asks ontological questions, builds deterministic models, and engages in the conduct of laboratory or bench science. The empiricist, on the other hand, asks epistemological questions and offers probabilistic models; outcomes research is thus a prominent form of medical empiricism.[26] To simplify, deterministic medical thinking organizes case-specific information around cause and effect; physician A observing symptom Z calls up the mechanism that is thought to produce it and acts accordingly. Probabilistic medicine eschews the question of why, organizing information around the likelihood of events; physician A observing symptom Z calls up the odds that treatment B will effect relief and acts accordingly.

Rival schools of medical science—and their respective bodies of medical knowledge—strain the logic of the applied-science model of medical care: which science is the conscientious practitioner expected to apply? Furthermore, either approach to medical decision making may rely more or less heavily on research results as opposed to, say, personal experience or the counsel of peers. Ironically for the outcomes movement, empiricism is especially susceptible to the influence of a physician's past experience, because probabilistic findings, however rigorous, are only of likely effectiveness over large populations. The physician is still left to figure the odds for a specific patient and determine if, in this case, they are odds worth taking. Evidence suggests that clinicians calculate "subjective probabilities," based on recollection of their own experience, to bridge this inferential gap.[27]

Purveyors of standard accountability claim to have done the hard work of finding facts. Theoretically, at least, their standards express the "evidence" and the "whole truth," and this usually means the findings of large statistical studies. The history of medical science and what we know about how physicians actually reason, however, raise several questions about the feasibility of erecting and promulgating such standards. For one, is the truest fact the most general or the most specific? Put differently, is relevance or rigor more characteristic of truth? How rigorous, moreover, is the rigorous collection and use of statistical evidence when it necessarily entails preanalytic delineation of subjects and variables? A recurrent dispute within medical empiricism[28] opposes studies of rigorously analyzable categories that merely approximate a patient's circumstances, to findings from methodologically compromised categories corresponding more directly to the particularities of illness and care. Which evidence compels the accountable physician, and by what logic is she to choose between them?

Both randomized controlled trials (RCTs) and outcomes research advance medical empiricism through the statistical analysis of patient-level data. RCTs, however, require rigor before relevance, while outcomes research makes methodological compromises to acquire information about day-to-day medical practice. To ensure the validity of their statistical analysis, RCTs typically collect new data from a carefully screened and randomly assigned study population. Outcomes research, in contrast, offers wider-ranging information more quickly by working with automated claims or other readily available data and the most practicable analytic methods. One reason for creating AHCPR as a separate, outcomes-oriented agency was reportedly the painstaking slowness and relative ungeneralizability of the National Institutes of Health's fastidious clinical trials.[29] Nevertheless, the experience of the first AHCPR-funded investigators (called Patient Outcomes Research Teams [PORT] I) prompted more stringent methodological requirements for studies funded in round 2. The PORT II studies are methodologically more like (but still different from) RCTs, not least because those who would speak science to uncertainty want to be certain, first, about their statistics.[30]

In any event, the trade-off of rigor and relevance receives attention primarily from a small number of methodologists, statisticians, and funding agencies. The broader outcomes movement and other sponsors of standard accountability, including most participants in the public discussion of accountability in health care, focus on the desirability of measurement per se, as if methodological dispute as to the validity of one measurement or another were merely an arcane and a temporary inconvenience. The scale of the health care enterprise and the development of ingenious techniques for measuring it seem to overshadow the conceptual refinement that would make actual research results more enlightening.

In fact, the very concept of outcomes is so variously defined as to include almost anything. For example, which are the meaningful surgery outcomes: health status at discharge, health status six months later, patient satisfaction, health status relative to cost? If all of them, how shall we weight their relative importance? When does an outcome evince effectiveness: when a patient is cured, when he is functional, when she is satisfied, when he is better off than he would otherwise have been, when she is not as well off as she might have been but is somewhat better off and has spent less than she might have; when one patient is better off, when all are, when the chances are 51 percent that all patients will be? And when do we really know what works: when we have one new and rigorous study, one rigorous but dated study, multiple studies of uneven quality, some evidence of a strong relationship, considerable evidence of a tentative relationship? Presumably there are good answers to many of these questions, especially from particular normative perspectives. Having committed themselves to a positivist conception of science, however, purveyors of standard accountability reject the inevitably normative basis for setting the terms of the research they champion.

Outcomes measurement is also beset by more mundane methodological problems. Are the right data, accurately and uniformly reported, readily available in sufficient numbers? Even if they are, how does the methodologist adjust for the extraneous effects of comorbidity, severity of illness, and patient preference? What outcomes will not be studied because the data are problematic, and at what point does the cost of the research outweigh its benefit? In some instances, outcomes studies have been found to be methodologically questionable years after research was completed and policy implications drawn.[31] The small-area variation researchers, for example, whose startling findings were an impetus to the new accountability, appear now to have chosen statistical methods that significantly inflated the size of the reported effects.[32] Questionable also is outcomes reporting wherein providers may improve their performance ratings by reworking the data. This seems to have been the case in New York State, where the Department of Health began to generate, from provider data, physician-specific mortality statistics for cardiac surgery. Although the risk-adjusted mortality rate for patients undergoing coronary artery bypass grafting declined in the first three years of reporting, 41 percent of the decline can be attributed to apparently spurious increases in patient risk factors. In other words, hospitals seem suddenly to be admitting much sicker patients, so the statistical performance of their physicians has automatically improved.[33]

Standard accountability, in summary, may be said to suffer from an insufficiency of truth—from an insistence on a single way of knowing that entails, but does not account for, normative assumptions, methodological conundra, and the delegitimation of much of what physicians seem really to know about their patients. Communicative accountability, in contrast, takes a pluralistic view of medical truth and requires physicians to represent a case as fully as possible. This includes the (correct) use of outcome studies and other kinds of probabilistic research, but always in combination with other kinds of knowledge, such as (well-understood) pathophysiological theory and bench science, (current) professional consensus statements, the physician's (considered) professional experience with other patients, (discerning) attention to the communicated experiences of colleagues, and (skilled) narrative negotiation with the patient. Possible outcomes are delineated, collaboratively, for the individual case, and outcomes research results are used if and when they apply. Unlike accountability based on statistics, communicative accountability does not flee particularization but demands it; physicians are accountable for the care of individual patients, and although aggregate probabilities may be informative, they do not to provide cover for an inattentive clinician. The truth criterion for communicative accountability demands a rigorous independence from a single source of evidence. Standard accountability, on the other hand, sacrifices the messy truth of clinical medicine to a superficially tidy presentation of selected evidence.

Truthful Uncertainty and Right Relations

In the communicative conception of physician accountability, the second and third functions of the physician's account are to state the limits of his representation and to establish a relationship where doctor-patient communication is the rule. Because standard accountability concerns itself with these functions only to a limited extent, the two approaches continue to diverge.

Perhaps most prominently, communicative accountability admits to medical uncertainty. Physicians do and will always treat patients under conditions of uncertainty.[34] Neither the most conclusive research findings nor the most intimate doctor-patient relationship eliminates the fundamental uncertainty of treating this illness, in this patient, at this time. Furthermore, clinical medicine is an inferential process that commonly operates without the benefit of complete information.[35] Practicing physicians accommodate this uncertainty as a matter of course. Although applied-science models equate technical rationality with medical rationality, actual physician decision-making evinces a highly rational and nontechnical reason, including professional judgment by individual doctors in specific situations.[36] The physician's "personal knowledge,"[37] which may be experiential and even sensory,[38] joins the available formal knowledge to the individual case. These eclectic data are organized through inference and intuition[39] by an independent, but not arbitrary or mystical, clinician. She deliberates rather than calculates, iteratively generating hypotheses to structure further data collection and interpreting data to refine hypotheses as a case evolves.[40] This internalized and continuous rationality predisposes the physician to, among other things, ongoing self-correction—not by conforming to some external standard but by what Donald Schon calls "reflecting-in-action"[41] on the fit between a case in progress and the progressively more complete understanding of it. At some point, sufficient understanding exists to support a confident clinical recommendation.[42] This in turn creates a new opportunity to engage the inevitable uncertainty of patient care.

Standard accountability also recognizes physician uncertainty but purports to diminish, if not eliminate, it. Health services researchers contend that substantial, undesirable, and unnecessary medical uncertainty is to blame for high rates of variation in the utilization of health services and is almost certainly wasteful, if not actually harmful, to patients. An uncertain physician will inappropriately take his cues from the local medical culture or the relevant reimbursement system, it is argued. "Making medicine more scientific,"[43] on the other hand, will improve significantly patient care, establishing "what works" and providing physicians with the definitive cue. Standard accountability also assumes the potential for certainty in how physicians think, that is, in the analytic regimens by which practitioners diagnose and treat. Algorithms and practice guidelines purport to distill the best thinking from point A to point B, and the introduction of Bayesian reasoning and decision analysis aims to replace the sloppy and subjective thought processes of the average physician with a disciplined, scientific approach to clinical choices. Even these technical advances would seem to leave room for uncertainty, however. Neither Bayes's rule nor decision analysis will, for example, ensure that the physician has begun with the right set of assumptions.[44]

Oddly enough, standard accountability eschews the individuality of communicative accountability even while the former makes recourse to physicians' self-justifying narrative at critical junctures. Physician profiling, for example, often entails first the use of statistical methods to identify physician "outliers," and then communication between the profiler and the outliers wherein errant physicians make justificatory accounts of their practice patterns. Similar procedures characterize utilization review and medical-board complaint processes. In other words, notwithstanding the establishment, legitimation, and violation of a standard, standard accountability eventually manifests itself in direct communication with the physician in question. This verbal account is then presumably evaluated for coherence, cogency, persuasiveness, and other narrative qualities by an interlocutor whose judgment is much like the clinical judgment of the physician under review. More fundamentally, practice guidelines are necessarily implemented by physicians, however willing, who must still decide—from a position outside the rules—that a given situation calls for a given guideline.

In sum, standard accountability privileges certainty, equating it, more often than not, with the product of probabilistic research. It posits that clinical uncertainty may be an unfortunate fact of life, at least at present, but it merely constrains truth and truthfulness; it does not define them. Communicative accountability, in contrast, not only admits to clinical uncertainty but is in fact achieved only to the extent that a physician weaves together the unknown and the known. The truth of an account may reside in its evidence—deterministic and probabilistic, objective and subjective, explicit and intuited—but its truthfulness is the physician's communicated awareness of the limits of this truth.

Finally, both standard and communicative accountability entail a relationship between physician and patient (or patient proxy such as payer or regulator). Under the standard conception, the physician-patient relationship is directed, almost entirely, toward criteria established before (and often outside) the clinical encounter. The accountable physician, then, relates to her patient in a way that will bring about those specific ends, and the exchange of information between physician and patient has been singled out as contributory to high levels of standard accountability. As noted previously, positivist social scientists credit physician-patient communication with improving patient outcomes, and to the extent that patients communicate their standards to be met, this exchange is the basis for all that follows. Although standard accountability increasingly relies on probabilistic research, when findings are equivocal about the desirability of one course over another, physicians must inform patients of their (equally effective) options, and patients must communicate to physicians their resultant choices. A case in point is John Wennberg, arguably the founder of the outcomes movement, who has recently argued for patient empowerment by means of computer software that informs and structures patients' decision-making processes.[45] Similarly, a recent outcomes study of the treatment of angina recommends that because patients have highly variable preferences for some outcomes over others, practice guidelines ought to be stratified by personal preference as well as severity of illness.[46]

Communicative accountability also entails the exchange of information, but here the quality of the exchange determines the usefulness of the information. In other words, whereas standard accountability requires physician-patient communication to move "data" from here to there, communicative accountability posits a physician-patient relationship wherein the meanings of illness and medical care are negotiated and renegotiated. The rightness of the relationship corresponds to its capacity for this important work—the time available, the mutual respect between participants, and other conditions for true collaboration, different perhaps in different relationships but always responsive to the particular combination of physician and patient.

In contrast to the scientism of standard accountability, communicative accountability does not purport to transcend particular clinical contexts. The physician, as well as the patient, then, may be—indeed must be—forthcoming about the influences on his conduct in any particular case. For the physician, these influences are increasingly political, as well as professional or cognitive. The era of medical outcomes is also the era of health care system reorganization; the fortunes of clinical medicine are in flux. Most notably, the expansion of managed care arrangements means that physicians are more often fiscally or organizationally constrained in the care they offer. Furthermore, in some quarters, the physician's role has been fundamentally redefined from that of treating individual patients to that of caring for whole communities.[47] This new physician is a steward of collective resources and will necessarily view any one patient as competitive with his neighbors—individually and as a group. Especially under these and other nontraditional medical economies, physician accountability ought to include disclosure and discussion of impinging resource allocation criteria.

Of course, novel economic arrangements are only one influence on patient care. Although standard accountability seems to imagine that the best rules will become the only rules, communicative accountability assumes that medicine will remain rife with ideals and obligations of various kinds. The medical profession, like every profession, inculcates adherence to the expressed norms of the group, and physicians are legally bound to standards of practice under medical-malpractice laws. Professional and personal ethics also shape the conduct of practitioners, and even under fee-for-service medicine, demands of payers and managers on behalf of their institutions may not serve individual patients, especially economically or socially marginal ones. Physician-patient collaboration must be self-conscious about these complex and crosscutting obligations and able to admit to and accommodate their influence on the case at hand.

Of course, physicians and patients are not equal parties to medical care. Although their collaboration is essential to communicative accountability, it is not to be mistaken for the collaboration of equals. Even under managed health care, physicians wield substantial power over their patients and substantially more power than their patients over the resources of the health care system. Nevertheless, physicians may act as "powerful, knowledgeable friends,"[48] who despite their knowledge and power (or because of it) understand accountability as communicative and communication as the act of two willing subjects. The communicative techniques for an accountable medicine are numerous, teachable, but ultimately idiosyncratic to individual relationships. The centrality of the account does not vary, however. Its negotiated meaning is the standard to which even standard accountability must answer.

Conclusion: Operationalizing Communicative Accountability

From the perspective of standard accountability, communicative accountability may seem utopian, or at least highly impractical. It does not lend itself to measurement, standardization, or the oversight of payers and managers. It does not promise certainty or hint at cost containment. Yet the case for communicative accountability derives from what we know of clinical medicine and is consonant with recent thinking in medical social sciences, humanities, and ethics. Moreover, as I have argued, the Habermasian criteria of truth, truthfulness, and rightness in communicative action are easily transposable to the accountability of physician to patient.

This proposal for communicative accountability is admittedly only a start—an argument for skepticism about the popular equation of accountability with research-based, quantifiable standards. It surely would benefit from follow-up studies of actual clinical accounts, on the one hand, and of implemented regimens of standard accountability, on the other. In what kinds of physician-patient relationships is accounting a collaborative act? To what extent do physicians distinguish truth from truthfulness? Under what circumstances do physicians disclose economic or organizational constraints on their practice? How do patients understand accounts based on probabilistic research? How do these accounts change, if at all, once a patient challenges the outcomes of his own care? What happens across settings of care, reimbursement systems, and nationalities?

With or without standard accountability's statistical methods, physicians and patients will pursue, more or less self-consciously, an intersubjective account of the illness that brings them together. Why not, then, increase physician accountability by specifying these three goals for the making of medical accounts: truth, truthfulness, and rightness? Far from utopian, there are at least four ways in which communicative accountability is more practical—as well as more accountable—than standard accountability.

First, the terms of communicative accountability are more immediately meaningful to patients. The average patient can judge and, most important, talk about whether the illness narrative is true, whether the physician is being truthful, whether the relationship with the physician is right. These are judgments that patients make and recount every day in relationships with other people. Furthermore, truth, truthfulness, and rightness are familiar enough concepts both to draw the patient into the clinical encounter and to organize her complaints against the physician should she seek redress outside the physician-patient relationship. Truth, truthfulness, and rightness are far more meaningful than the statistical terms of evaluation for evidence (significance, confidence interval, standard deviation, meta-analysis) or for individuals (probabilities of outcomes or risk statistics).

Second, to the extent that accountability in health care is accountability to the patient's own standards, truth, truthfulness, and rightness are more substantive than the ubiquitous "patient satisfaction." Whether or not satisfaction predicts future service utilization, it is a blunt instrument for advancing accountability to patients, especially those who are "dissatisfied" or "partially satisfied" with the current accounting for their illness and care. Specifying their dissatisfactions as related to truth, truthfulness, or rightness at least provides recognizable structure for the "careful conversation"—structure for both the patients' grievances and the physicians' responses.

Third, communicative accountability makes the physician the accountable party and means it. This allows her to choose, and requires her to explain, whatever outside standard is admitted into the clinical encounter. Especially in the U.S. health care system, there is rarely a single practice guideline for a given condition; rather, professional organizations, government agencies, research institutes, payers, and managed care organizations all produce standards to which physicians may be held. How, then, is adherence to one of these standards in and of itself an act of accountability? Is it not, in fact, the very opposite—submergence of the individual account in an aggregate norm? What recourse is there, then, for a patient on the wrong side of probability, one whose treatment by the rules leaves him unwell and unsettled. He is unlikely to secure an accounting from AHCPR or the American College of Physicians. Rather, this is the physician's role, and communicative accountability makes it unambiguous.

Finally, communicative accountability, by being forthright about uncertainty and influence, invites patients, as patients, members, policyholders, and citizens, to participate in their care and in the health care system. Would it not improve the quality of the next health care reform debate if citizens understood the conditions of their medical care not through abstraction or ideology but as narrators of their own health policy stories and as seekers after truth, truthfulness, and rightness in the stories of others?

In 1987 John Stoeckle wrote, "That new modes of relationships through personal communications, new attachments, or changes in doctors' behaviors and explanations of illness might also improve treatment is an entirely uncommon thought." This proposal for communicative accountability has tried to make more common the thought that some new modes—not entirely new, but sorely underdeveloped and recently out of favor—would indeed improve physicians' accountability to the patients they treat.

NOTES

1. "Health Care in Crisis: Wasted Health Care Dollars," *Consumer Reports* 57 (1992): 435–88; J. F. Fries et al., "Reducing Health Care Costs by Reducing the Need and Demand for Medical Services," *NEJM* 329 (1993): 321–5; M. J. Mehlman, "Health Care Cost Containment and Medical Technology: A Critique of Waste Theory," *Case Western Reserve Law Review* 35 (1986): 778–877.

2. A. S. Relman, "Assessment and Accountability: The Third Revolution in Medical Care," *NEJM* 319 (1988): 1220–2.

3. A. M. Epstein, "The Outcomes Movement—Will It Get Us Where We Want to Go?" *NEJM* 323 (1990): 266–9.

4. S. J. Tanenbaum, "What Physicians Know," *NEJM* 329 (1993): 1268–71; S. J. Tanenbaum, "Knowing and Acting in Medical Practice: The Epistemological Politics of Outcomes Research," *Journal of Health Politics, Policy, and Law* 19 (1994): 27–44.

5. J. Habermas, "What is Universal Pragmatics?" in *Communication and the Evolution of Society*, trans. T. McCarthy (Boston: Beacon Press, 1979), pp. 1–68.

6. D. M. Frankford, "The Critical Potential of the Common Law Tradition," *Columbia Law Review* 94 (1994): 1076–123.

7. Habermas, "What is Universal Pragmatics?", p. 33.

8. Habermas, "What is Universal Pragmatics?", p. 33.

9. L. M. L. Ong et al., "Doctor-Patient Communication: A Review of the Literature," *Social Science and Medicine* 40 (1995): 903–18.

10. K. M. Hunter, *Doctors' Stories: The Narrative Structure of Medical Knowledge* (Princeton: Princeton University Press, 1991).

11. M. Good, *American Medicine: The Quest for Competence* (Berkeley: University of California Press, 1995), p. 199.

12. R. Charon et al., "Literature and Medicine: Contributions to Clinical Practice," *Annals of Internal Medicine* 122 (1995): 599–606.

13. B. Good and M. Good, "The Meaning of Symptoms: A Cultural Hermeneutic Model for Clinical Practice," in *The Relevance for Social Science in Medicine*, ed. L. Eisenberg and A. Kleinman, (Dordrecht, The Netherlands: Reide, 1981), pp. 165–96.

14. A. Kleinman, *The Illness Narratives: Suffering, Healing, and the Human Condition* (New York: Basic, 1988).

15. Charon et al., *Literature and Medicine,* p. 602.

16. E. Haavi Morreim, *Balancing Act: The New Medical Ethics of Medicine's New Economics* (Washington, D.C.: Georgetown University Press, 1995), p. 146.

17. Morreim, *Balancing Act,* p. 147.

18. P. M. Ellwood, "Outcomes Management: A Technology of Patient Experience," *NEJM* 318 (1988): 1549–56.

19. J. E. Wennberg, "Dealing with Medical Practice Variations: A Proposal for Action," *Health Affairs* 3 (1984): 6–32; D. M. Eddy, "Variations in Physician Practice: The Role of Uncertainty," *Health Affairs* 3 (1984): 74–89.

20. C. Anderson, "Measuring What Works in Health Care," *Science* 263 (1994): 1080, 1082.

21. J. E. Sisk and S. A. Glied, "Innovation under Federal Health Care Reform," *Health Affairs* 13 (1994): 82–97.

22. F. Davidoff, K. Case, and P. W. Fried, "Evidence-Based Medicine: Why All the Fuss?" *Annals of Internal Medicine* 122 (1995): 727.

23. Davidoff, Case, and Fried, "Evidence-Based Medicine."

24. H. R. Wulff et al., *Philosophy of Medicine: An Introduction* (Oxford: Blackwell Scientific Publications, 1990); D. R. Gordon, "Clinical Science and Clinical Expertise: Changing Boundaries between Art and Science in Medicine," in *Biomedicine Examined*, ed. M. Lock and D. Gordon (Dordrecht: Kluwer, 1988), pp. 257–95.

25. Tanenbaum, "Knowing and Acting"; R. A. Kreisberg, "An Abundance of Options," *NEJM* 329 (1993): 413–6.

26. Wulff et al., *Philosophy of Medicine*.

27. Tanenbaum, "Knowing and Acting"; Wulff et al., *Philosophy of Medicine*.

28. Anderson, "Measuring What Works", pp. 1080, 1082.

29. Anderson, "Measuring What Works".

30. Anderson, "Measuring What Works".

31. Anderson, "Measuring What Works".

32. M. Schwartz et al., "Small Area Variations in Hospitalization: How Much You See Depends on How You Look," *Medical Care* 32 (1994): 202–13.

33. J. Green and N. Wintfeld, "Report Cards on Cardiac Surgeons: Assessing New York State's Approach," *NEJM* 332 (1995): 1229–32.

34. E. B. Beresford, "Uncertainty and the Shaping of Medical Decisions," *Hastings Center Report* 21 (1991): 6–11; S. Gorovitz and A. MacIntyre, "Toward a Theory of Medical Fallibility," *Journal of Medicine and Philosophy* 1 (1976): 51–71.

35. J. Kassirer, "Teaching-Problem Solving—How Are We Doing?" *NEJM* 332 (1995), no. 22: 1507–9.

36. A. S. Elstein et al., *Medical Problem-Solving: An Analysis of Clinical Reasoning* (Cambridge: Harvard University Press, 1978); G. J. Groenand and V. L. Patel, "Medical Problem-Solving: Some Questionable Assumptions," *Medical Education* 19 (1985): 95–100; M. W. Wartofsky, "Clinical Judgment, Expert Programs, and Cognitive Style: A Counter-Essay in the Logic of Diagnosis," *Journal of Medicine and Philosophy* 11 (1986): 81–92.

37. M. Polanyi and H. Prosch, *Meaning* (Chicago: University of Chicago Press, 1975).

38. Tanenbaum, "Knowing and Acting"; Gordon, "Clinical Science".

39. Wartofsky, "Clinical Judgment"; H. L. Dreyfus and S. E. Dreyfus, *Mind over Machine: The Power of Human Intuition and Expertise in the Era of the Computer* (New York: Free Press, 1986).

40. Kassirer, "Teaching-Problem Solving".

41. D. A. Schon, *The Reflective Practitioner: How Professionals Think in Action* (New York: Basic 1983).

42. Kassirer, "Teaching-Problem Solving".

43. H. Hiatt and L. Goldman, "Making Medicine More Scientific," *Nature* 371 (1994): 100.

44. Kassirer, "Teaching-Problem Solving".

45. J. E. Wennberg, "Innovation and the Policies of Limits in a Changing Health Care Economy," in *Technology and Health Care in an Era of Limits*, ed. A. C. Gelijns (Washington, D.C.: National Academy Press, 1992), pp. 3–33.

46. R. F. Nease et al., "Variation in Patient Utilities for Outcomes of the Management of Chronic Stable Angina: Implications for Clinical Practice Guidelines," *JAMA* 273 (1995): 1185–90.

47. M. R. Greenlick, "Educating Physicians for the Twenty-First Century," *Academic Medicine* 70 (1995): 179–85.

48. Morreim, *Balancing Act*, p. 146.

Contributors

Susan E. Bell, Ph.D., is in the Department of Sociology and Anthropology at Bowdoin College

Philip J. Boyle, Ph.D., is Senior Vice-President and Editor at The Park Ridge Center

Daniel Callahan, Ph.D., is Director of International Programs at The Hastings Center

Larry Culpepper, M.D., M.P.H., is Professor of Family Medicine at Memorial Hospital of Rhode Island/Brown University

Paul J. Edelson, M.D., is Chairman of Pediatrics at New York Methodist Hospital

Fred Gifford, Ph.D., is in the Philosophy Department at Michigan State University

Ruth S. Hanft, Ph.D., is in the Department of Health Services Management and Policy at George Washington University

Susan E. Kelly, Ph.D., is a Research Fellow at the Stanford University Center for Biomedical Ethics

Barbara A. Koenig, Ph.D., is Executive Director of the Stanford University Center for Biomedical Ethics

Donald J. Murphy, M.D., is Regional Medical Director at GeriMed of America, Inc., in Denver.

James Lindemann Nelson, Ph.D., is in the Department of Philosophy at the University of Tennessee

Pieter F. de Vries Robbé, is on the Faculty of Medical Sciences at Katholieke Universiteit Nijmegen, the Netherlands

Judith Wilson Ross, M.A., is an Associate at the Center for Health Care Ethics of the St. Joseph Health System

Jane Sisk, Ph.D., is a Professor in the Division of Health Policy and Management of the School of Public Health at Columbia University

Sandra J. Tanenbaum, Ph.D., is Professor of Health Policies at Ohio State University

Gert Jan van der Wilt, is on the Faculty of Medical Sciences at Katholieke Universiteit Nijmegen, the Netherlands

Robert M. Veatch, Ph.D., is Professor of Medical Ethics at the Kennedy Institute of Ethics at Georgetown University

Dick Willems, M.D., is a physician in the Netherlands

Index

Accountability, communicative
   assumptions of, 218
   contrast to standard accountability, 208–11
   in health care, 205
   justification for, 207
   operationalizing, 218–20
   physician/patient relationship, 217
   truth in, 214
Accountability, standard
   argument for, 211
   certainty with, 216
   contrast to communicative accountability, 208–11
   physician/patient relationship, 217
   physician's role in, 205
   truth in, 214
Agency for Health Care Policy and Research (AHCPR)
   Clinical Practice Guidelines, 181
   evidence of OME panel, 78–80
   factors in guideline priorities, 72–73
   glue ear guideline, 94
   guideline panel composition, 76–78
   methods to produce guidelines, 78
   outcomes research and practice guidelines of, 208–9
   ownership of OME guideline, 82–83
   Patient Outcome Research Teams (PORT), 25
   practice guidelines, 60–67, 71
   selection of guideline topics, 73–74
Aging
   medicalization of, 115

American College of Physicians (ACP)
   guidelines for hormone therapy, 117–18
   practice guidelines, 49–54
American Medical Association (AMA)
   technology assessment initiative, 23
Aristotle, 200
Autologous Blood and Bone Marrow Transplant Registry-North America, 133

Bias
   in outcomes data, 171–72
   suspicion of, 7–10, 92
Biomedical model
   disease in, 119
   lack of quality of life focus in, 121
Bone marrow transplantion (BMT), 133
Breast cancer
   advocacy groups, 143–44
   social factors in HDC/ASCR for, 135–37
British Thoracic Society, 155

Cancer treatment
   BMT as treatment for diffuse, 133
   HDC/ASCR, 128–29
Cardiopulmonary resuscitation (CPR), 103
Cataract surgery
   process in creating RAND practice guidelines, 56–57
   RAND literature review, 55–56

Chemotherapy, high-dose
  for breast cancer, 126–27
  rescue after, 126
Clinical judgment
  defined, 196
  distinct from outcomes research and practice guidelines, 199–200
  as physicians' justification, 11–13
  physicians' reliance on experience, 11–13
  in practice, 169–70, 202
  response to knowledge sources, 198
Clinical trials
  AIDS, 143
  bilateral OME, 92–94
  Framingham longitudinal, 22
  HDC/ASCR, 140
  outcomes data from, 153
  post-World War II public and private, 22
Clinicians. See Physicians.
Communication, human (Habermas), 206
Comprehensive Health Planning Act (1974), 22
Consensus conferences
  areas covered, 189
  NIH Office of Medical Applications of Research (OMAR), 189
  NIH ovarian cancer screening, 44–49
Cost-effectiveness analysis
  used by AHCPR OME panel, 80

Data
  AHCPR otitis media with effusion guideline, 62
  American College of Physicians guideline, 51–54
  effect of absent research data, 42–43
  for experimental technologies, 131–32
  interpretation of, 112
  NIH Consensus Conference, 44–49
  physician concern related to, 8–10
  RAND Corporation cataract surgery guidelines, 55–56
  statistical significance, 173–74
  See also Outcomes data
Databases, computerized, 24
Development process
  AHCPR otitis media guidelines, 72
  for practice guidelines, 71–72
Diagnosis Related Groups (DRGs), 24–25
Dreyfus, Hubert, 200

Estrogen, 113–14
Evidence
  AHCPR panel development and evaluation of, 78–80
  in practice guidelines and treatment protocols, 183–86
Expert opinion, 167

Facts
  distinct from values, 189–90
  in standard accountability, 211–12
Feyerabend, P. K., 190
Fleck, Ludwig, 190
France
  implementation of guidelines, 157–59
  practice guideline development, 154

Glue ear
  epidemiology and natural history of, 86–87
  treatment (1860–1960), 87–88

Glue ear, *continued*
  treatment effects, 89–90
  treatment (1960 to present), 88–89
Good, Mary-Jo D., 207
Grady, Deborah, 117
Great Britain
  development of practice guidelines, 155
  implementation and outcome of guidelines, 159–60
Guidelines
  AHCPR otitis media with effusion, 60–68, 80–83
  American College of Physicians Counseling for Menopausal Women, 49–54, 67–68
  authoritative, 42–44, 67–68
  for developing guidelines, 107
  development and production of, 42, 68, 71
  NIH Consensus Conference on Ovarian Cancer, 44–49, 67–68
  RAND cataract surgery, 54–60, 67–68
  to rationalize medical practice, 43–44
  related to influence of money, 104–6
  related to treatment of otitis media, 72–83
  See also Practice guidelines

Habermas, Jürgen, 205–6
HDC/ASCR. *See* High-dose chemotherapy/autologous stem cell rescue (HDC/ASCR).
Health care costs
  as issue (1970s), 22
  relation of technology to, 22–23
Health maintenance organizations (HMOs)
  implementation of outcomes research and guidelines, 27–28
  making outcomes/technology assessment decisions, 27
Hematopoietic growth factors, 133
High-dose chemotherapy/autologous stem cell rescue (HDC/ASCR)
  conflicts related to, 129–30
  contested meanings of, 145–46
  as controversial treatment, 137
  effects on patients receiving, 134–35
  formal assessments of, 140
  local assessment of data, 139–40
  popularizing mechanism for, 144
  procedure, 133–34
  uses of, 128–29
Hormone therapy
  meta-analysis in asymptomatic postmenopausal women, 116–20
  social and cultural context, 115–16
  to treat menopausal symptoms, 111–14

Individualism
  related to clinical practice, 138–39
  related to value of technology, 138
Information
  in communicative accountability, 217
Institute of Medicine (IOM), 72
Insurance companies
  implementation of outcomes research and guidelines, 27–28
  response to HDC/ASCR therapies, 141–43
Interest groups
  AIDS activists, 143
  breast cancer advocacy, 143–44
  for HDC/ASCR, 143–44

Judgment
  clinical, 201–2
  ethical, 200

Judgment, *continued*
    expert, 200–202
    of physicians, 196–97

King's Fund Centre, Great Britain, 155
Knowledge, scientific, 112–13, 130–31
Kuhn, Thomas, 190

Legislation
    Comprehensive Health Planning Act, 22
    related to guideline development, 71–73
    Women's Health Equity Act, 143
Lerner, Debra, 121
Levine, Sol, 121
Lewis, Sinclair, 3
Liability, legal, 14–15
Literature review
    AHCPR practice guidelines, 61–62
    American College of Physicians, 50–52
    RAND Corporation, 55–56
Luckmann, Thomas, 190

Malpractice, 106–7
Managed care organizations, 26
Measurements
    physicians' use of, 100–101
    questions about, 101–2
    reporting, 103
    reporting risk reductions, 104
    sources of information for, 103
Medicaid program
    Oregon experiment, 25–26, 28
    payment for patients in managed care, 26
Medical necessity concept, 23, 26–27

Medical practice
    clinical judgment in, 202
    in communicative accountability, 205–7
    construction of link to outcomes data, 161–62
    guidelines to rationalize, 43–44
    interventions using technology assessment for decisions for, 111
    outcomes research related to, 24
    practice guidelines in, 41
    practice pattern variation, 31
    relation to technology assessment, 111–21
    social factors related to HDC in, 135–37
    uncertainty in, 111
    using guidelines to change, 42
    See also Practice guidelines
Medical review
    criteria of AHCPR OME panel, 83–84
    development of measures for, 83–84
Medicare program
    under AHCPR guidelines, 73
    change in payment to hospitals (1983), 24–25
    high costs of, 22, 25
    medical necessity concept under, 23, 26–27
    outcomes data collection proposal, 26
Menopause
    focus of studies related to, 120
    medicalization of, 115, 120
    use of hormone therapy to treat symptoms, 111–14
Meta-analysis
    American College of Physicians literature review, 51–52
    described, 117
    of hormone therapy, 116–20

Meta-analysis, *continued*
  as technology assessment, 112–13
  translation to clinical guidelines, 121
Money
  influence on medicine, 104–6

National Academy of Sciences, Institute of Medicine Council on Health Care Technology, 24
National Agency for the Development of Evaluation in Medicine (ANDEM), France, 154, 157
National Center for Health Care Technology (NCHCT), 23, 24
National Institutes of Health (NIH)
  Consensus Conference on Ovarian Cancer screening, 44–49
  Consensus Development Conferences, 181–82
  Office of Medical Applications of Research (OMAR), 189
  selection of guideline topics, 74–75
Naturalism, 137–38
Netherlands, the
  development of practice guidelines in, 155–57
  implementation and outcome of guidelines, 158–60

Office of Medical Applications of Research (OMAR). *See* National Institutes of Health (NIH).
Office of Technology Assessment (OTA), 22
Otitis media
  acute, 73–74
  guideline development process, 73
Otitis media with effusion (OME)
  alternative treatment modes, 90–91
  as focus of panel, 74
  treatment effects, 89–90
Outcomes
  concept of, 213
  consideration by AHCPR OME panel, 80–81
  measurement of, 214
  negotiation of scientific, 112
Outcomes data
  biased or value laden, 171–72
  construction of link to practice, 161–62
  differences from practice guidelines, 168–69
  generation of, 5
  obstacles to use of, 6–16
  outcomes research based on, 167
  physicians' moral concerns related to, 4
  physicians' response to recommendations of, 11–14
  practice guidelines based on, 167
  skepticism related to, 6–8
  sources of, 153
  translated into practice guidelines, 153
Outcomes movement, 15, 103, 208, 213
Outcomes research, 167
  of AHCPR, 208
  development, 24
  epistemic stance in, 198
  goals for, 28–29
  implications of changes in philosophy of science, 191
  practice guidelines based on, 198, 202
  used in communicative accountability, 214
  using meta-analysis, 24
  what is provided by, 192–93
  See also Patient Outcomes Research Team (PORT)

232 Index

Panels
   composition, 76–78
   expertise, 75–78
   focus and outcome of OME panel, 78–83
Patient Outcomes Research Team (PORT)
   studies, 187
   as use of technology assessment, 181
Patient preferences
   AHCPR otitis media with effusion guideline, 65
   American College of Physicians guideline, 53
   measurement of, 103
   NIH Consensus Conference, 48–49
   as part of practice guidelines, 48–49
   physician concern related to, 10–11
   RAND Corporation cataract surgery guidelines, 59
Patients
   concept of individualized care of, 32–35
   perception of physician judgment, 197
   resistance to practice guidelines and treatment protocols, 193
   See also Physician/patient relationship
Performance standards, AHCPR OME panel, 83–84
Pharmaceutical companies, 116
Philosophy of medicine
   epistemic stance in, 198–99
   on role of technology assessment, 189–90
Philosophy of science
   incorporation of judgments, 190
   paradigm in, 190
   post-Kuhnian, 190–91
   on role of technology assessment, 189–90

Physician/patient relationship
   therapeutic importance, 33–35
   trust in, 103
   See also Patient preferences
Physicians
   under communicative accountability, 205, 210–11, 214–15
   compliance with guidelines, 100
   conditions for disregard of practice guidelines, 167–68
   effect of guideline development on practice, 139–40
   factors in compliance with guidelines, 100
   financial incentives for, 104–6
   judgment of, 196–7
   legal liability concerns, 14
   moral concerns of, 4–6, 10–13
   objections related to outcomes studies, 7–18
   ranking of practice guidelines, 71
   resistance to practice guidelines and treatment protocols, 193
   resistance to recommendations associated with outcomes, 11–18
   skepticism about outcomes data, 6–10
   under standard accountability, 209–10
   theoretical structure of clinical decisions, 182–83
   under threat of malpractice, 106–7
   treatment of patients under uncertainty, 215–16
   use of guidelines, 198
   use of measurements in diagnosis, 100–101
   view of patient preferences, 10
Practice guidelines
   Agency for Health Care Policy and Research, 60–67
   of AHCPR, 209

Practice guidelines, *continued*
  American College of Physicians, 49–54
  authority of NIH Consensus Conference on ovarian cancer, 49
  based on outcomes data, 167
  conditions affecting valid recommendations, 71
  development and implementation in France, 154, 157–59
  development and implementation in Great Britain, 155, 159
  development and implementation in the Netherlands, 155–57, 158–59
  differences from outcomes data, 168–69
  expressing authority, 42–44
  function of, 181, 183–87
  from outcomes research, 153, 202
  patient preferences of NIH Consensus, 48–49
  physicians' criticism of, 167–68
  physician skepticism of, 6–8
  problems and limitations of, 161–62
  process of development, 5, 71–72
  RAND Corporation, 54–60
  resistance to, 193
Preferences. *See* Patient preferences.
Progestin treatment, 114

Quality assessment, AHCPR OME panel, 83–84
Quality of life
  effect of hormone therapy on, 118
  recommended for studies of menopause, 120–21

RAND Corporation practice guidelines, 54–60
Reasoning, explicit, 169–70

Resource allocation
  decision making in national health plans, 29
  in democratic societies, 29
  at federal level, 28
Risk stratification, 102

Science
  negotiation and consensus in, 112
  voice of lifeworld in, 120–21
  See also Philosophy of science.
Statistical analysis
  elements of, 170–78
  meta-analysis, 21
  for risk stratification, 102
Statistical analysis. *See* Data; Outcomes data.
Stem cell rescue, 133–34

TA. *See* Technology assessment.
Tanenbaum, Sandra, 35, 198–99, 201
Technology
  assessment and adoption of medical, 127–28
  experimental, 126–29, 132–35
Technology assessment
  cultural assumptions, 145–46
  for experimental technologies, 127–29
  federal level, 24–25
  function of, 180–82
  legitimate factors in, 128
  local, 129–30
  in making medical decisions, 111
  in a market economy, 29–30
  meta-analysis as method of, 117
  in philosophies of science and medicine, 189–90
  pre-1970s period, 21–22
  private sector initiatives, 23–25

Technology assessment, *continued*
  public sector focus, 23–26
  social context of, 130–32
  1970s period, 22
  use of medical technologies, 127
  value judgments in, 193
Treatment protocols
  function of, 181, 183–87
  resistance to, 193
Trust
  in physician/patient relationship, 103
Truth
  in standard accountability, 214

Uncertainty
  under communicative and standard accountability, 215–18
  in medical practice, 41, 111
  of physicians, 5–6
  role of risk stratification in reducing, 102–4

U.S. Preventive Services Task Force, 75–76
Utilization review, 209

Value judgments
  in practice guidelines and treatment protocols, 183–87
  relation to facts, 189–90
Values
  distinct from facts, 189–90
  hidden in outcomes data and practice guidelines, 8–10
  role in medical science, 191–92

Women
  decision making related to breast cancer, 144–45
  menopausal and postmenopausal, 111–16
Women's Health Equity Act, 143